Other Harvard Medical School books published
by Simon & Schuster

*Harvard Medical School Family Health Guide*
Harvard Medical School

*Six Steps to Increased Fertility*
Robert L. Barbieri, M.D., Alice D. Domar, Ph.D.,
and Kevin R. Loughlin, M.D.

*The Arthritis Action Program*
Michael E. Weinblatt, M.D.

*Healthy Women, Healthy Lives*
Susan E. Hankinson, Sc.D., Graham A. Colditz, M.D.,
JoAnn E. Manson, M.D., and Frank E. Speizer, M.D.

*Eat, Drink, and Be Healthy*
Walter C. Willett, M.D.

*The Aging Eye*
Harvard Medical School

A Harvard Medical School Book

# The Sensitive Gut

Fireside

New York   London   Toronto   Sydney   Singapore

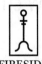

FIRESIDE
Rockefeller Center
1230 Avenue of the Americas
New York, NY 10020

Copyright © 2000, 2001 by the President and Fellows of Harvard College
Illustrations copyright © 1999 by Harriet Greenfield

FIRESIDE and colophon are registered trademarks
of Simon & Schuster, Inc.

For information about special discounts for bulk purchases,
please contact Simon & Schuster Special Sales:
1-800-456-6798 or business@simonandschuster.com

Designed by William P. Ruoto

Manufactured in the United States of America

1  3  5  7  9  10  8  6  4  2

Library of Congress Cataloging-in-Publication Data
Lasalandra, Michael.
The sensitive gut / [written by] Michael Lasalandra and
Lawrence S. Friedman.
p.   cm.
"A Harvard Medical School Book."
Includes bibliographical references and index.
1. Intestines—Diseases—Popular works.
I. Friedman, Lawrence S.   II. Title.
RC860.L373 2001
616.3'4—dc21                              2001050153
ISBN 0-7432-1504-4

This publication contains the opinions and ideas of its author. It is intended to provide helpful and informative material on the subjects addressed in the publication. It is sold with the understanding that the author and publisher are not engaged in rendering medical, health, or any other kind of personal professional services in the book. The reader should consult his or her medical, health, or other competent professional before adopting any of the suggestions in this book or drawing inferences from it.

The author and publisher specifically disclaim all responsibility for any liability, loss, or risk, personal or otherwise, which is incurred as a consequence, directly or indirectly, of the use and application of any of the contents of this book.

Harvard Medical School gratefully acknowledges Michael Lasalandra, the writer of this work, and Lawrence S. Friedman, M.D., Professor of Medicine at Harvard Medical School and Physician at the Gastrointestinal Unit of Massachusetts General Hospital, our faculty consultant.

# Contents

# The
# Sensitive
# Gut

# Introduction

*You can't ignore the importance of a good digestion. The joy of life . . .
depends on a sound stomach, whereas a bad digestion inclines one to
skepticism, incredulity, breeds black fancies and thoughts of death.*
—Joseph Conrad, *Under Western Eyes*

You wouldn't think that the seemingly simple task of eating a meal could cause so many difficulties. Yet this source of so much pleasure—and so many nutrients that are vital to our health—is frequently responsible for myriad intestinal complaints from a large portion of the world's population.

Painful stomach cramps, a gnawing discomfort in the abdomen, a burning sensation behind the breastbone, an uncomfortable feeling of fullness, belching, bloating, nausea, embarrassing gas, diarrhea, constipation—these can all be the consequences of our love affair with food.

Sometimes these miseries can occur without our ever taking a bite. It is well known that stress—brought on by a job interview, a college exam, an important decision at work, a date, a doctor's appointment, even a family reunion—can send our stomachs on an unpleasant roller-coaster ride.

Everyone from prince to pauper has been known to suffer one or more of these stomach-related indignities from time to time. Studies show that some complaints reportedly occur frequently in up to one-quarter to one-half of the world's population.

For most of us, such intestinal upsets are infrequent and relatively tolerable, such as when they are the consequence of an intestinal bug, a trip to a foreign land, or a gluttonous holiday meal. But one in four people has frequent gastrointestinal problems that can severely disrupt a normal lifestyle. Sufferers often endure uncomfortable and unnecessary medical tests, spend a king's ransom on questionable cures, and miss countless days of work.

Though the misery they inflict is real, these problems are considered "functional" gastrointestinal (GI) disorders—that is, they usually cannot be attributed to an infection or physiological abnormality, unlike ulcers or stomach cancer, for example. There is no medical explanation for the complaints of more than 20 percent of the people who consult a gastroenterologist. Just because doctors cannot find an organic cause (that is, an identifiable structural, biochemical, or infective basis for complaints), however, patients should not blame themselves for their problems or assume the problems are imaginary. The symptoms—the stomach discomfort, bloating, feelings of fullness, belching, and burning—are real.

Despite medicine's frustrations and limitations in these areas, people plagued by GI distress definitely can be helped. This book focuses on a number of disorders considered functional: gastroesophageal reflux disease (GERD), functional dyspepsia, irritable bowel syndrome (IBS), constipation, diarrhea, and excessive gas.

Although these maladies sound different in name, sometimes the problems they cause are similar and symptoms overlap. And despite their serious-sounding names, these disorders usually do not imply serious illness. Still, if they occur frequently or last more than a month, most people so afflicted will seek help.

While there is, unfortunately, no tried-and-true cure for a sensitive gut, help is available. People plagued by gastrointestinal distress can benefit from a better understanding of their symptoms. With proper knowledge, and the support of a thoughtful, caring doctor, people can worry less and focus on dietary and lifestyle changes that can relieve symptoms—or at least make coping with them easier.

# 1

# How the Gut Works

*A good set of bowels is worth more to a man than any
quantity of brains.*
—Henry Wheeler Shaw

*Gut.* It's an ancient Anglo-Saxon word that refers to the
human digestive system. Think of this marvel of nature's engineering as a perpetual food processor, constantly
mixing, grinding, and transforming into biologically useful
molecules the meats, vegetables, fruits, and snacks that we
put into our mouths three times a day or more.

Nearly thirty feet long if stretched out flat, the gut is a
chain of hollow organs linked in a long, twisting tube that
runs from the mouth to the anus and includes the esophagus (or gullet), the stomach, small intestine, colon, and rectum. This string of organs is also known as the alimentary
canal or gastrointestinal tract.

These organs break down food and liquids—carbohydrates, fats, and proteins—into chemical components that
the body can absorb as nutrients and use for energy or to
build or repair cells. What's left is expelled by a highly effi-
cient disposal system.

The gut is a dynamic organ that is almost always moving, driven by the muscle in its walls. This muscle consists of an outer longitudinal layer and an inner circular layer. In a process resembling a hydraulic system, the coordinated contractions of these layers move the intestinal contents along. Muscles within the walls contract and relax, pushing food and fluids through the length of the canal, in much the same way as rolling waves deposit sand and shells on the shore. This dynamic movement along the gastrointestinal tract is known as peristalsis.

Helping the job of digestion get done is the mucosa, or lining, of the mouth, stomach, and small intestine, which harbors glands that produce digestive enzymes. The salivary glands, liver, and pancreas also secrete juices that similarly help in turning food into soluble material that can be easily absorbed into the bloodstream (see Figure 1.1).

The entire process is coordinated and controlled by a remarkable network known as the enteric nervous system (ENS), an intricate nerve complex in the gut wall that communicates with the brain via the spinal cord. The ENS, in turn, is influenced by hormones, neurotransmitters, and connections to the central nervous system (including the vagus nerve and the sympathetic nerve fibers that emanate from the spinal cord) that affect muscle, mucosa, and blood vessels in the digestive tract. The ENS communicates with the brain, first via the sympathetic nerves that pass to and from the gut through transformers called sympathetic ganglia. These nerves connect to the spinal cord and then to the base of the brain. In addition, parasympathetic nerves link with the base of the brain via the vagus nerve from the upper gut or the sacral nerves from the colon. Each nerve transmission is imparted by one of several neurotransmitters or hormones acting upon a suitable receptor in muscles or in nerve ganglia. The gut-brain system, scientists say, is nearly equal in complexity to the body's central nervous system.

The brain and gut are intricately intertwined—but you already knew that. It's painfully obvious to most of us, judg-

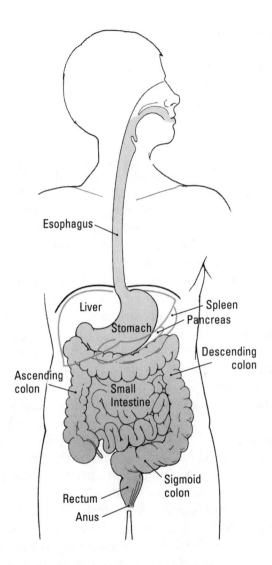

## FIGURE 1.1: THE GASTROINTESTINAL TRACT

The digestive tract consists of the esophagus, stomach, small intestine, colon, rectum, and anus. The mucosa—or surface layer of cells lining the mouth, stomach, and small intestine—contains tiny glands that produce digestive enzymes. The liver and pancreas, which are connected to the digestive tract, also secrete juices that help break down food into soluble products that can be absorbed into the bloodstream.

ing by how emotional events can cause our guts to churn and do flip-flops that can be nearly as discomforting to us as those caused by foods that don't agree with us or bugs picked up in foreign lands.

## The Digestive Journey

Pop a grape, a cherry tomato, or a succulent shrimp into your mouth. Immediately, digestion begins. In the mouth itself, the tongue and teeth help to get the process started by chewing and chopping the food so that it is small enough to be swallowed. The chewing process, as well as the carbohydrates in the foods we eat, prompt the salivary glands to secrete saliva, which contains an enzyme called amylase that starts changing some starches into simple sugars and softening the food to additionally aid in the swallowing process. The saliva also allows the taste buds of the tongue to sense the flavors of our foods—where would the enjoyment be if we couldn't distinguish and sense the variety of flavors that make eating such a pleasurable activity?

Swallowing is actually a very complicated, coordinated act that begins with the tongue pushing food back into our throat, or pharynx. This voluntary action sets off an involuntary chain of events that transports the food from the throat through the esophagus and into the stomach, a journey that typically takes eight seconds.

Food does not simply drop down this passageway by means of gravity. If it did, how would astronauts eat? No, you can actually eat and drink while standing on your head, although it would probably take some getting used to. Things move through the esophagus because they are pushed by contractions of the esophageal muscles. Whether the stomach is up or down doesn't matter.

Think of the esophagus (and entire intestine, for that matter) as an empty tube surrounded by coats of muscles that contract in a succession of waves. As the ball of food—called a bolus—reaches the far end of the sixteen-inch-long esophageal tube, the lower esophageal sphincter (LES) opens to allow the food to exit, then closes again. This muscular tube is quite elastic; it can stretch to nearly two inches across to accommodate foods of various sizes.

While the esophagus is moving things along, it also must keep things from backing up or regurgitating and reentering the throat. That's where the other gatekeeper—the upper esophageal sphincter—comes into play. The two sphincters, upper and lower, make sure the food moves in the proper direction.

Control of these complex actions is activated by the swallowing center of the brain. In the course of normal swallowing, the brain sends messages ahead, relaxing the LES even before the food arrives, so that the trapdoor is open and ready.

Occasionally, though, things can go wrong.

The LES keeps food from being forced from the stomach back up into the esophagus, but if it relaxes too often or for too long a time, or is weak to begin with, sometimes gastric acid washes back, or refluxes, into the gullet, causing what is commonly known as heartburn.

If the esophagus is a tube or passageway with valves at both ends, the stomach can be thought of as a warehouse, a storage facility, where the food can be prepared for digestion. This food warehouse is an accommodating place that can hold a little afternoon snack or expand to comfortably handle a five-course meal. On average, the stomach holds from one to one and a half quarts—but records exist showing stomachs with an amazing six-quart capacity. If the stomach did not have this huge storage capacity, we'd have to eat frequent small meals and we'd be unable to drink large quantities of liquids at any given time. To use its great storage capacity, the stomach must relax its muscles. If it doesn't, we may feel uncomfortable or bloated.

The stomach doesn't just hold food, however; the muscles in the lower stomach also mix the food into a soft mush. This mixing is aided by the liquids we drink, by saliva, and by hydrochloric acid and the enzyme pepsin, both of which are produced by the glands that line the stomach. Hydrochloric acid and pepsin help to break down proteins into their basic parts, amino acids. After all of this mixing, our once-palatable meal is reduced into a thick liquid called chyme. Just why the stomach's potent hydrochloric acid doesn't dissolve stomach tissue is a mystery; the stomach mucosa clearly has some sort of defense system to protect itself.

The other important function of the stomach, after storing and then grinding and mashing the food, is to deliver the resulting chyme to the small intestine in amounts that can be handled; too large a load could overwhelm the intestine's ability to absorb nutrients. Peristaltic contractions in the stomach drive this mixture through the pyloric sphincter a muscular gate, into the duodenum, the first part of the small intestine (see Figure 1.2). The process of delivering chyme to the intestine occurs over time and is affected by numerous factors—a variety of hormones, what's been ingested (fluids move more quickly than solids), and external considerations, emotions, and physical exercise. All can either delay or stimulate gastric emptying.

The stomach is a specialized muscle designed to push its contents along by a series of involuntary contractions governed by nerves connecting the stomach wall to the brain via spinal cord. The nerves that carry impulses from the gastrointestinal (GI) tract are called visceral nerves. While the somatic nerves on the surface of the abdomen can feel various stimuli such as heat, cold, and pressure, the visceral nerves inside the stomach and intestines recognize only stretching, pulling, or expansion (distension) of the muscles of the intestinal wall. When the stretching, pulling, or expansion are excessive, pain can result.

When we have not eaten for a while and our stomach is

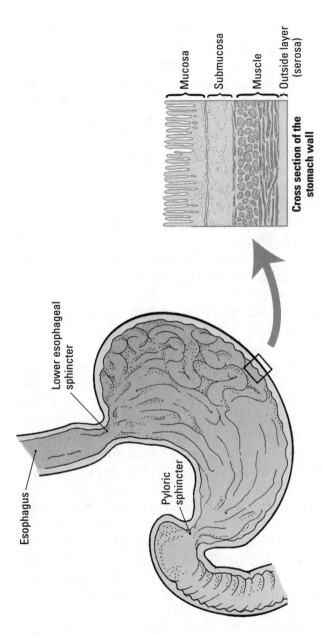

**FIGURE 1.2: A CLOSE-UP OF THE STOMACH**

Swallowed food travels to the stomach via the esophagus and passes through the lower esophagus and then through the lower esophageal sphincter. Glands in the stomach lining produce digestive juices, and muscles in the lower stomach wall churn and mash foodstuffs into liquid. Muscle contractions drive this mixture through the pyloric sphincter into the duodenum.

empty, the stomach initiates a series of rhythmic contractions known as hunger pangs. They serve as a signal to the brain: "Feed me!" These contractions also explain stomach noises, which may be caused when air and fluid are rattling around inside us. Sometimes we may feel cramping as contractions intensify, relax, and then intensify again. If the contractions are sudden and severe, we feel what are known as spasms. These disturbances in the patterns of stomach (and intestinal) contractions may result from disturbances in the electrical impulses that are designed to regulate the motor activity of the stomach.

After accepting a typical meal, it takes about two hours for the muscular stomach to reduce our food to a liquid and have it ready to move along to the small intestine. A high-protein meal can take an extra hour or two. A high-fat meal can take up to six hours.

The small intestine, which includes the duodenum, jejunum, and ileum and is actually about twenty-one feet long, is the next stop on our food's journey through the digestive tract. The main work of digestion—the process of breaking down fats, starches, and proteins into amino acids, fatty acids, and simple sugars and absorbing them—takes place here in this long tube as food is bathed in digestive enzymes and secretions from the liver and pancreas. Most liquids move through the small intestine within an hour, while solids take about three to five hours. Fats and proteins take the longest to move.

To begin, the stomach empties food through the pyloric sphincter into the foot-long duodenum, located a few inches above the navel. Many minerals, such as iron and calcium, are absorbed through the cells lining the duodenum. Also here, bile and pancreatic juices are added to the mix. Bile, produced by the liver and stored in the gall bladder, emulsifies fats for easier processing. Pancreatic enzymes, such as trypsin, amylase, and lipase help digest proteins, carbohydrates, and fats. In the second portion of the small intestine, the jejunum, which measures eight feet in length, fats, starches, and proteins are broken down and absorbed by the lining cells as the chyme moves along as if on a conveyor belt. In the third and lowest portion of the small intestine, the ileum—twelve feet in length—water is absorbed, along with vitamin $B_{12}$ and bile salts.

Reduced to products that the body can manage, nutrients from digested food are absorbed by the intestine's thin lining and sent to cells throughout the body via the bloodstream and lymphatic system.

Finally, the remaining unused or unusable material arrives in the colon, or large intestine, a four-foot-long muscular tube about the diameter of your fist, the walls of which act like a sponge and soak up 80 to 90 percent of the water still present. In fact, the colon absorbs about a quart of liquid from material it receives from the ileum each day. Inside the colon, food residue travels up the right side and across the transverse colon, descends on the left side (behind the stomach), passes through the sigmoid colon to the rectum (behind the left groin), and exits. It can take anywhere from four to seventy-two hours for food to move through the colon.

Bacteria that reside in the colon help in the digestive process by feeding off whatever remains of our meals—the glycoproteins and carbohydrates not absorbed in the small intestine. The bacteria also produce hydrogen, carbon dioxide, and methane gas, as well as fatty acids, which provide energy for cells lining the colon.

Undigested or undigestible matter, such as fiber, is propelled distally, or forward, away from the center of the body, by contractions of the colon wall and settles as solids in the rectum—the final foot or so of the colon. The rectum is guarded by a sphincter muscle at the anus that helps control defecation, or the release of this waste. The waste accumulates until the rectal wall becomes so distended that it signals the internal anal sphincter to relax, triggering an urge for a bowel movement, and tells us it is time to go to the bathroom. Fortunately, the external anal sphincter, which is under voluntary control, keeps the rectal contents in place until defecation can be carried out at a convenient, socially acceptable time. What comes out is primarily water and colon bacteria, plus bile, mucus, and cells normally shed from the intestinal lining. Undigested food makes up very little of the average one-quarter- to one-half-pound stool. Nature does not waste food.

When all goes according to nature's plan, this long, complex process—which can take anywhere from eighteen hours to several days from eating a meal to eliminating it—is something we hardly think about.

But when something goes wrong—when the gut acts up—it can cause us untold miseries.

# 2

# Gastroesophageal Reflux Disease

You enjoyed the meal—but now you're paying for it, big time. You've got an uncomfortable burning sensation radiating up through the middle of your chest. It can hit after eating spicy foods, but it's not always associated with eating—it can come when you lie down to take a nap, or each night at bedtime, too. Many women experience this sensation during pregnancy, most commonly in the later stages.

Sometimes the pain is so intense that a person fears he or she may be having a heart attack. But in most cases, they are simply experiencing heartburn, the most common gastrointestinal malady.

An estimated one-third of Americans experience heartburn at least once a month, with 10 percent feeling the burn nearly every day. A recent survey of 1,000 sufferers by the American Gastroenterological Association revealed that 65 percent of sufferers experience heartburn both during the day and at night, with 75 percent saying the problem keeps them from sleeping at night and 40 percent saying that nighttime heartburn affects their job performance the next day. This heartburn epidemic leads us to spend nearly $2 billion a year on over-the-counter antacids alone. It is clearly a major problem.

Heartburn is the major symptom of a condition known as gastroesophageal reflux disease (GERD), a phenomenon in which acid and pepsin rise from the stomach into the esophagus, much like water bubbling up into a sink from a plugged drain.

The burning sensation is usually felt in the chest just below the breastbone, though it often extends from the root of the neck to the lower end of the chest cage. It can persist for hours and may be accompanied by brief rushes of highly acidic fluid into the back of the throat that causes a very unpleasant stinging sensation. It can also be accompanied by a sour taste in the mouth.

It is the burning behind the sternum that is at the heart of heartburn. A variety of foods, certain emotions, such as anger or fear, and even particular positions, like reclining or bending forward, can aggravate the condition.

While heartburn is certainly a nuisance to millions of people, others seem to live with it quite well. Usually, it is not a sign of serious illness, but simply another bit of evidence that we humans are not designed perfectly. Still, many people spend countless hours and untold billions of dollars looking for a way to spell relief.

## Causes of Reflux

Gastroesophageal reflux disease is a digestive disorder that affects the lower esophageal sphincter (LES), the muscle connecting the esophagus with the stomach. The LES is a high-pressure zone that acts as a barrier to protect the esophagus from the backflow of gastric acid from the stomach.

The LES is a complex segment of smooth muscle under the control of nerves and various hormones. Normally, it works something like a dam, opening to allow food to pass into the stomach and closing to prevent food and acidic stomach juices from flowing back into the esophagus. If the LES loses its tone, however, it cannot close up completely after food empties into the stomach. Gastroesophageal reflux occurs in just such a situation, when the LES is weak or relaxes inappropriately and allows the stomach's contents to flow up into the esophagus (*see* Figure 2.1). Scientists aren't sure exactly why this happens, though it is known that dietary substances, drugs, and nervous-system factors can impair its function.

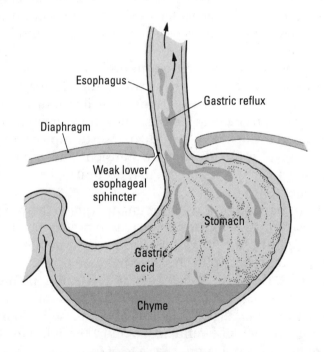

**FIGURE 2.1: GASTROESOPHAGEAL REFLUX**

Gastroesophageal reflux occurs when the lower esophageal sphincter, a high-pressure zone designed to keep digestive juices in the stomach, relaxes more than it should. When this happens, gastric acid refluxes into the esophagus, causing heartburn.

Other factors besides malfunctions of the LES contribute to reflux as well. In one study, about one-half of GERD patients exhibited abnormal nerve or muscle function in the stomach that caused impaired motility—an inability of the stomach muscles to contract in a normal fashion. The result may be a delay in the emptying of the stomach, which increases the risk that acid will reflux back into the esophagus: acid remains at the "top" of the stomach, near the LES, rather than moving downward, adding to both pressure on the LES and the likelihood of reflux. A failure of peristaltic contractions to clear the esophagus of acid that has refluxed, an impaired ability of the esophageal lining to resist refluxed acid, or a shortage of saliva (which has a neutralizing effect on acid) may all factor into heartburn too.

Episodes of reflux often go unnoticed, but when they are excessive, the gastric acid irritates the esophagus and may produce the pain experienced as heartburn. Sometimes acid regurgitates as far as the mouth and may come up forcefully as vomit or as a "wet burp." Most symptoms of gastroesophageal reflux disease are transient and occur only after a big meal; symptoms also may occur if a person bends over or lies down.

Overweight people and pregnant women may suffer more heartburn spells because increased pressure in the abdomens contributes to reflux. Pregnant women are also more prone to heartburn because increased progesterone levels relax the LES. Weight lifters also suffer plenty of heartburn; excessive bending and lifting, abdominal exercises, girdles, and tight belts can all increase abdominal pressure and provoke reflux. Generally, though, GERD is uncommon in people under the age of forty.

Still, diet and lifestyle habits can contribute to LES dysfunction in people of any age. Smoking, for instance, can irritate the entire gastrointestinal tract. Frequent sucking on a cigarette causes air to be swallowed, increasing stomach pressure and encouraging reflux. The smoke itself may also irritate the delicate lining of the digestive tract. Smoking sometimes also relaxes the LES muscles. Alcohol, too, can irritate the esophageal lining and loosen the lower esophageal sphincter, as can coffee and other products containing caffeine. Coffee, tea, cocoa, and cola drinks are also all powerful stimulants of gastric acids, so they can pack a double punch. And mints and chocolate—often served to cap off a meal, presumably to aid in digestion—can actually make things worse. Each relaxes the LES and may thereby induce heartburn.

Fried and fatty foods in general contribute to heartburn in many people. Some people say that onions and garlic give them heartburn. Citrus fruits and tomato products are cited by others. The bottom line is that if you notice that a particular food seems to lead to episodes of heartburn, by all means stay away from those foods. Thus, for many people with frequent heartburn, staying away from deli meats, hot dogs, mustard, and Indian, Mexican, Szechuan, and other spicy cuisines is probably a good idea.

How you eat, however, can be as important as what you eat. Skipping breakfast or lunch and then consuming a huge meal at day's end can increase gastric pressure and the possibility of reflux. And lying down right after eating will only make the problem worse. It is best to wait three hours after eating a meal before going to bed—and stay away from late-night snacks, too.

Finally, even a modest weight gain may increase the abdominal pressure that can induce heartburn, so a low-fat diet is a good idea for more than just one reason. Exercise can help in the battle of the bulge and, as such, may help moderate the effects of heartburn and GERD. Exercise can also help relieve stress, and that can ease symptoms too. However, some types of exercise, such as running and the aforementioned weight lifting, may bring on heartburn symptoms.

Many heartburn sufferers—and even their doctors—may be unaware that some prescription drugs can exacerbate heartburn. Oral contraceptives or postmenopausal hormone preparations containing progesterone are known culprits, as are aspirin and other nonsteroidal anti-inflammatory drugs (NSAIDs). Corticosteroid drugs, commonly used to treat asthma, rheumatoid arthritis, multiple sclerosis, and other illnesses are known to cause heartburn. In addition, certain drugs such as alendronate (Fosamax), used to treat osteoporosis, may irritate the esophagus. And some antidepressants, tranquilizers, calcium-channel blockers, and the asthma medication theophylline can relax the LES, thereby contributing to reflux. *(See* Chart 2.1, Medications That May Cause or Worsen Gastroesophageal Reflux.)

Other medical conditions may also contribute to GERD. About one-half of asthma patients suffer from reflux, though it is not clear whether asthma is a cause or effect of GERD. Some experts speculate that the coughing that accompanies an asthma attack may cause pressure changes in the chest that trigger reflux. Asthma medications containing theophylline, which dilate the airway, may also relax the LES and contribute to GERD. Other illnesses that may contribute to GERD include diabetes, peptic ulcers, and some types of cancer.

GERD, in fact, is a little-known but frequent complication of more severe cases of diabetes, related, perhaps, to the slow emptying of the stomach associated with diabetic neuropathy. GERD may also be caused by peptic ulcers and gastric cancer, as both can obstruct the stomach and prevent gastric acid from flowing distally, thereby allowing the acid to back up into the esophagus. In most such cases, however, symptoms of the ulcer or cancer—such as upper-abdominal pain and weight loss—overshadow those of GERD. Furthermore, cancer treatments such as chemotherapy, as well as narcotics used to manage pain, may also give rise to problems with gastric motility.

# CHART 2.1: MEDICATIONS THAT MAY CAUSE OR WORSEN GASTROESOPHAGEAL REFLUX

| GENERIC NAME | BRAND NAME | USE |
|---|---|---|
| **Bronchodilators***<br>theophylline | Accurbon, Aerolate, Aquaphylin, etc. | Relieve wheezing |
| **Calcium–Channel Blockers***<br>diltiazem<br>nifedipine<br>verapamil | Cardizem<br>Adalat, Procardia<br>Calan, Isoptin | Lower blood pressure and improve coronary artery blood flow |
| **Nonsteroidal Antiinflammatory Drugs (NSAIDs)***<br>aspirin<br>ibuprofen<br>naproxen | Bufferin, Ecotrin, and others<br>Advil, Motrin<br>Aleve | Relieve pain and inflammation |
| **Osteoporosis Drug***<br>alendronate | Fosamax | Builds bone and reduces risk of fractures |
| **Progestins***<br>medroxyprogesterone acetate<br>norethindrone acetate | Amen, Provera<br>Aygestin, Norlutate | Relieve symptoms of menopause; used in oral contraceptives |
| **Tricyclic Antidepressants***<br>amitriptyline<br>nortriptyline<br>protriptyline | Elavil, Endep<br>Pamelor<br>Vivactil | Relieve depression; occasionally used for chronic pain |

* Not all available drugs are listed.

## The Hiatal Hernia Connection

For years, debate has raged among medical researchers over the possible connection between reflux disease and hiatal hernia, a common condition in which part of the stomach protrudes into the chest cavity through a hiatus, or opening, in the diaphragm, the muscle that separates the chest and abdomen and helps with breathing *(see* Figure 2.2). Some studies indicate that a hiatal hernia may be the result of a lack of fiber in the diet.

A hiatal hernia is a weakness in the diaphragm that allows a protrusion of the stomach above the diaphragm. This changes the angle at which the esophagus joins the stomach, softens the ligaments that hold these organs together and in proper alignment, and inhibits the LES's ability to prevent reflux. Recent studies indicate that hiatal hernia results in retention of acid and other stomach contents above the opening in the diaphragm. These substances can reflux easily into the esophagus.

While many people with small hiatal hernias (hiatus less than three centimeters) exhibit no symptoms, others report significant heartburn discomfort. Almost all people with large hiatal hernias (hiatus greater than three centimeters) experience reflux. And hiatal hernias are almost always present in people with GERD who have moderate to severe esophagitis, or inflammation of the esophagus. So, although hiatal hernias and reflux occur independently, there is support for the idea that the two conditions are related.

Hiatal hernias may exist in up to 30 percent of the population—and in most people past retirement age. In the 1960s, doctors went out of their way to find hiatal hernias and repair them surgically. In subsequent years, as the prevailing view came to be that GERD and hiatal hernia were merely coincidental, surgery to repair hiatal hernias has

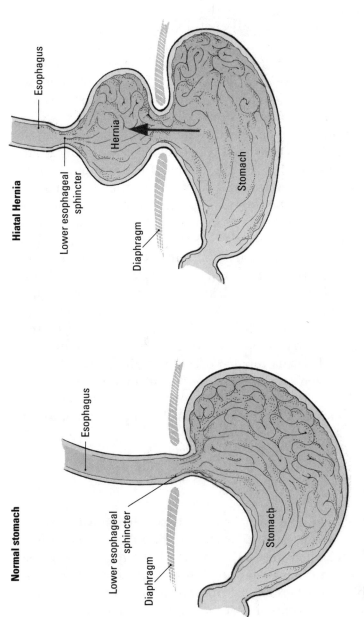

**Normal stomach**

Esophagus

Lower esophageal sphincter

Diaphragm

Stomach

**Hiatal Hernia**

Esophagus

Lower esophageal sphincter

Hernia

Diaphragm

Stomach

### FIGURE 2.2  HIATAL HERNIA

Hiatal hernia is a condition in which part of the stomach protrudes upward into the chest through an opening in the diaphragm, the band of muscle that separates the chest from the abdomen.

dropped off. Today, we find that the truth seems to lie somewhere in between—that hiatal hernias sometimes may impair LES activity and sometimes may not. In any case, surgical repair of hiatal hernias is much less common now that more effective drug therapies, including proton-pump inhibitors and histamine $H_2$-receptor antagonists, which suppress the secretion of stomach acids, exist.

Even so, treatment of hiatal hernias may be necessary if the hernia is so large that it is in danger of becoming strangulated—twisted in a way that cuts off blood supply—or is complicated by severe GERD or esophagitis. In instances such as these, the doctor may perform surgery to reduce the size of the hernia or to prevent strangulation. Operations for hiatal hernia to correct GERD are serious, but not difficult, and require entering the left chest cavity or the abdomen. Nowadays, the surgery can often be carried out through a laparoscope, a flexible tube with a camera at the tip that can be inserted through a tiny incision into the abdominal cavity. Narrow surgical tools can then be passed through the laparoscope. In the hands of a competent surgeon, hiatal hernia repair works very well. However, there can be problems with the operation. Recurrence of the hernia is always a possibility, and the operation can bring with it difficulties in swallowing, as well as bloating, if the sphincter muscles are made too tight.

## Diagnosing Reflux

Most people deal with heartburn on their own, without seeking medical care. That's how it should be. A doctor may be helpful when the symptoms worry the patient or if they interfere with day-to-day life, but for most people, it is reasonable to try to relieve symptoms without a doctor's intervention. Since one-third of the population has heartburn, a battery of tests on everyone is just not practical.

For those who do seek the help of a doctor, a detailed account of symptoms will help make the diagnosis.

A doctor will evaluate the patient's history and ask detailed questions about the nature of the pain and its pattern of onset. He or she will ask whether symptoms are worse after eating a heavy meal and whether they are associated with such known troublemakers as spicy or fatty foods, citrus fruits, onions, garlic, chocolate, coffee, or alcohol. The doctor will also want to know if bending over to tie shoelaces or lying down aggravates the symptoms and whether the pain can be linked to anxiety. Of further interest is whether regurgitated stomach contents leave a bitter or acidic taste in the mouth, or if the patient has experienced a sudden outpouring of salty fluid in the mouth, called water brash, which is produced by salivary secretions stimulated by reflux.

In the great majority of cases, a diagnosis of gastroesophageal reflux disease is straightforward, particularly if the patient gives a typical description of heartburn and acid regurgitation. In such a case, doctors usually forgo diagnostic tests and proceed right to treatment—usually starting with antacids and modifications in diet and lifestyle. If a patient obtains relief, particularly from antacids, the odds are that the diagnosis of GERD was correct.

One important issue to consider is that with chest pain, there's always the chance that the patient is suffering a heart attack. Symptoms associated with GERD can, in fact, mimic the pain of a myocardial infarction (heart attack), or angina (a temporary insufficiency of blood flow through the coronary arteries), especially when the sensation produced is constriction rather than burning in nature.

Thus, it can be dangerous to simply assume that your chest pain is caused by reflux. Yet even the best doctor can slip now and then in diagnosing chest pain—so if that's the case, how can you be sure that you are correct in self-diagnosing heartburn? The main thing is to try to judge the severity and length of your chest pain. If it is a severe pressing or squeezing discomfort, it may be a heart attack. And heart attack pain lasts. If your pain goes away in five or ten minutes, it is probably not a heart attack. It could be angina, however, and angina pain does require a visit to the doctor—and treatment.

It is important, then, not to dismiss angina-like chest tightness, especially if it follows physical exercise. And though this is serious, it may be comforting to know that when people who exhibit anginal symptoms are screened for coronary artery disease, nearly 30 percent have normal coronary arteries.

About 600,000 people come into emergency rooms each year complaining of chest pain. Roughly 100,000 of them are believed to have GERD. In some studies, reflux disease accounts for up to one-half of the cases of non-cardiac chest pain. Nevertheless, people with known reflux disease should always seek medical attention if they experience chest discomfort during or after exercise.

A trial of a relatively high dose of omeprazole, a drug that blocks stomach acid secretion, may help lessen the need for invasive tests to identify GERD in patients with chest pain. In one small study, eighteen of twenty-three patients who actually had GERD reported relief after seven days of taking omeprazole, whereas only two out of fourteen patients who did not have GERD symptoms experienced improvement.

Beyond the possibility of heart problems, frequent non-burning chest pain, bleeding into the gastrointestinal tract, dysphagia (difficulty in swallowing), hoarseness, or chronic coughing and wheezing may all be associated with GERD—but all also have other causes and tests that can help determine these causes (see box, Is This Test Necessary?).

Gastroesophageal reflux can cause such respiratory problems as asthmatic wheezing, coughing, or hoarseness. When asthma strikes adult nonsmokers with no history of

## IS THIS TEST NECESSARY?

Doctors ordinarily don't put heartburn patients through costly diagnostic evaluations. However, more serious reflux symptoms, such as bleeding from the esophagus or swallowing problems, may warrant further investigation. Common tests include the following:

☞ **Barium studies** In this procedure, the patient drinks a liquid barium sulfate mixture and then undergoes an X-ray examination of the chest and abdomen. The barium, a contrast medium, defines the upper gastrointestinal (GI) tract on the X-ray image and can help the physician identify problems such as hiatal hernias and esophageal lesions or strictures. This test has been the standard means to view the upper GI tract since the early twentieth century and is considered completely safe.

☞ **Upper GI endoscopy** Here, the physician inserts a flexible tube down the throat, having first sedated the patient and depressed the gag reflex with a local anesthetic spray. The tube contains a light and a camera that allow the doctor to carefully inspect the lining of the esophagus, stomach, and small intestine, assess injuries such as ulcers or strictures, and take a biopsy (tissue sample) if necessary. This procedure may be recommended for patients with severe and long-standing heartburn or difficulty swallowing, or for those who have a stricture or lesion identified via a barium study. The test is more expensive than a barium study and carries a small risk of bleeding or perforation of the esophagus, stomach, or small intestine.

Other tests for GERD that are performed less frequently include the following:

☞ **pH monitoring** This method monitors an individual's reflux episodes over twenty-four hours via a thin, acid-sensing probe inserted nasally and positioned just above the lower esophageal sphincter. The patient can eat, drink, and move about while the probe transmits data to a portable box worn around the waist. Although moderately expensive and somewhat uncomfortable, this test is the best method for documenting reflux in patients who have unexplained chest pain, coughing, wheezing, or hoarseness.

☞ **Bernstein test** Used—after a cardiac cause has been ruled out—to determine whether chest pain is related to reflux, this procedure involves the infusion of saline and then diluted hydrochloric acid into the esophagus through a nasal tube, to see if the acid reproduces the patient's pain. The test is particularly useful for patients with an "acid-sensitive" esophagus; that is, people who experience heartburn when even very small amounts of acid are refluxed into the esophagus. With the availability of more convenient, less uncomfortable pH studies, the Bernstein test is used less commonly now than in the past.

☞ **Esophageal manometry** In this test, thin catheters are inserted through the nose into the esophagus to measure the pressure within the esophagus and lower esophageal sphincter. Manometric results are helpful for selecting candidates for antireflux surgery and for detecting motility disorders (abnormal contractions of the esophagus) that may cause chest pain or swallowing difficulty. Although the patient must swallow a thin rubber tube, esophageal manometry is generally not too difficult to endure and is considered risk-free.

---

lung disease or allergies, reflux pH probe studies can identify whether GERD is the culprit.

Researchers speculate that when caustic acid refluxes into the esophagus, it triggers a nerve reflex that constricts the bronchial tubes (the branches of the trachea that lead into the lungs) and induces wheezing. Aspiration of acid into the bronchi may also play a role in causing these symptoms. On the other hand, it may be that asthma leads to gastroesophageal reflux and not vice versa. Only 10 percent of the population suffers from GERD, but 50 percent of people with asthma have GERD, a statistic that strongly suggests a connection. Coughing and wheezing create pressure shifts in the chest that can produce reflux; moreover, theophylline and other bronchodilators may weaken the LES.

## Beyond Heartburn

Though simple reflux is uncomfortable, it usually doesn't present any real danger to healthy individuals. One-half to nearly three-quarters of those with reflux disease have mild symptoms that are usually cleared up through simple measures. But if patients develop persistent gastroesophageal reflux disease and suffer frequent relapses, and their condition goes untreated, serious problems can develop over time.

These problems can include severe narrowing (stricture) of the esophagus, erosion of the lining of the esophagus, ulcers, precancerous changes in esophageal cells, and trouble with tooth decay and sleeping.

Narrowing, or stricture, of the esophagus may need to be dilated. This is done by way of endoscopy, using a balloon or special dilator to reopen the affected area. About one-third of patients who need this procedure require a series of dilation treatments to fully open the passageway.

Reflux esophagitis is an inflammation of the esophagus, caused by backflow of acid and pepsin from the stomach. The inflammation ranges in severity from redness to actual erosions of the mucosa, the surface layer of cells that line the esophagus. When such erosions occur, the condition is known as erosive esophagitis. In addition to the burning sensation of heartburn, patients with esophagitis may also complain of pain behind the breastbone spreading into the back or up into the neck, jaw, or even ears. This pain can be so intense that a sufferer may fear that he or she is having a heart attack. It may be accompanied by trouble swallowing; foods seem to stick in the throat before going down the gullet and hot drinks may be unpleasant to swallow. A patient may also have some acid fluid regurgitated into the throat, resulting in a cough; nausea is a symptom as well.

More aggressive inflammation of the esophagus may

also cause coughing and nausea, and may even lead to bleeding. Endoscopy or a barium study is usually used to confirm esophagitis and locate any strictures.

Treatment of active bleeding from ulcers in the inflamed esophagus may require blood transfusions and use of a probe passed through an endoscopic tube to apply electricity or heat to coagulate the blood and stop the bleeding.

Barrett's esophagus, another complication of chronic inflammation, is an abnormality in which the squamous, or flat, cells normally lining the lower esophagus are replaced by taller cells resembling those that line the stomach or intestine. The condition is caused by chronic and severe exposure to acid from the stomach and bile from the small intestine brought on by severe GERD. Barrett's esophagus can, over time, develop into cancer, so patients with this condition are urged to have regular endoscopic evaluations (including biopsies) to identify malignant changes as early as possible.

Barrett's esophagus, in fact, is a proven risk factor for cancer in the lining of the esophagus, a cancer that is appearing with increasing frequency in the United States. Still, it occurs in only a small number of all GERD patients. Persons most at risk are those—usually middle-aged white men—who developed GERD at an early age and have endured it for many years. For persons who develop cancer, surgery to remove the esophagus, often in combination with chemotherapy, is the standard treatment.

An experimental procedure called photodynamic therapy has also shown promise for removing early cancers and precancerous tissues in patients with Barrett's esophagus. Photodynamic therapy has been used successfully in the treatment of some lung cancers, and some doctors are trying it for treatment of Barrett's esophagus as well. The idea is to prevent premalignant cells from becoming cancerous. The treatment involves injecting a drug, aminolevulinic acid (ALA), which makes cells highly sensitive to light; only precancerous cells absorb the drug. Then, a laser probe activates the drug, causing it to produce a chemical that kills the abnormal cells. The treatment is still considered experimental and, although less invasive than surgery, can be accompanied by a number of unpleasant side effects.

A 1999 study by researchers at Sweden's Karolinska Institute has reported a higher risk for esophageal cancer in GERD patients, particularly those who have Barrett's esophagus. Some experts think that refluxed bile rather than acid may be a special risk factor for causing esophageal cancer.

Finally, GERD can result in dental and sleep problems. People who lose dental enamel, the hard substance covering teeth, absent any other risk factor (such as the chronic vomiting associated with bulimia, for example) may be able to attribute the problem to chronic reflux. Acid reflux may also cause spasms of the vocal cords or larynx that can block the flow of air to the lungs. One study has reported that these sorts of spasms may be at the root of sleep apnea, a condition in which breathing stops briefly but frequently during sleep. Patients suffering from sleep apnea are often drowsy during the day and are at increased risk for high blood pressure and even heart attacks.

## Self-Care

Modifying one's diet and lifestyle form the foundation for treating the symptoms of reflux. The basic idea is to prevent the problem by keeping the contents of your stomach in the stomach and staying away from foods that loosen the lower esophageal sphincter.

Here are some effective prevention tips for people troubled by heartburn. Following some or all of them may eliminate the problem or reduce the frequency or severity of flare-ups.

☞ **Graze, don't gorge.** Eat smaller meals and eat more slowly. Because a large meal will remain in the stomach for several hours and thereby increase the chances for gastro-esophageal reflux, those who suffer from the problem should distribute their food intake over three, four, or even five smaller meals over the course of the day.

☞ **Relax while you eat.** Stress increases the production of stomach acid, so make meals a pleasant, relaxing experience. Sit down. Eat slowly. Chew completely. Play soothing music.

☞ **Relax between meals.** Relaxation therapies such as deep breathing, meditation, massage, tai chi, and yoga may help relieve and prevent heartburn.

☞ **Remain upright after eating.** Postures that reduce the risk of reflux should be maintained for at least three hours after a meal. And avoid bending or straining to lift heavy objects during that period.

☞ **Avoid bedtime snacks.** Eat nothing within three hours before hitting the sack.

☞ **Lose weight.** Excess poundage increases pressure on the stomach and can push acid up into the esophagus. That's one of the reasons why so many pregnant women suffer from heartburn.

☞ **Loosen your belt.** Don't wear tight belts, waistbands, or other clothing that puts pressure on your stomach.

☞ **Avoid the burn foods.** Abstain from food and drink that increase acid secretions, decrease LES pressure, or slow stomach emptying. Known offenders include high-fat foods, spicy dishes, tomatoes and tomato products, citrus fruits, garlic, onions, milk, carbonated drinks, coffee (including decaf), tea, chocolate, mints, colas, and alcohol.

☞ **Snuff the butts.** Nicotine stimulates stomach acid and impairs LES function.

☞ **Chew gum.** Chewing gum can increase saliva production, soothing the esophagus and washing acid back down to the stomach.

☞ **Consult your pharmacist or doctor.** Drugs that can predispose you to reflux include aspirin, nonsteroidal anti-

inflammatory drugs, estrogen, narcotics, tricyclic antidepressants (such as amitriptyline), and asthma medications.
If a drug you take causes heartburn, ask your pharmacist or
doctor about an effective substitute.

☛ **Raise your head at night.** If you are bothered by nighttime heartburn, elevate the head of your bed by placing six-
inch blocks under its legs, or place a wedge under your
upper body. Don't try to elevate your head by sleeping on
extra pillows, however. That makes reflux worse by bending
you at the waist and compressing the stomach.

☛ **Exercise smartly.** Engage in vigorous physical activity
only after the stomach is empty, usually at least two hours
after eating a meal.

## Antireflux Drug Therapy

Most people have become aware of the most convenient
and least expensive reflux treatments thanks to the almost
nonstop television and radio advertisements promoting a
variety of antacids—pills, tablets, and liquids—that treat
heartburn by lessening the acidity of refluxed material. In
addition to antacids, some histamine $H_2$-receptor blockers
can be purchased over the counter. While they are generally
a little more effective than antacids, they cost a little more.
Newer GERD remedies called proton-pump inhibitors illus-
trate the old adage that you get what you pay for: these
by-prescription-only medications are superior therapies,
but don't come cheap. Some people find relief by using a
combination of these drugs or a variety of herbal remedies.

### Antacids

These cheap, over-the-counter remedies are effective in
neutralizing digestive acids in the stomach and esophagus,
at least in mild cases of heartburn. The best times to take any

antacid is after a meal or when symptoms occur. Many people find tablets more convenient, but liquids provide faster relief.

Antacids taken regularly can provide temporary or partial relief from reflux. However, there are so many on the market that choosing the best one can be confusing. Besides cost, it is important to consider a product's sodium content, acid-neutralizing power, possible reaction with other medications, and impact on other parts of the gastrointestinal (GI) tract. (*See* Appendix, Drugs Used to Treat Functional Gastrointestinal Disorders.)

There are three basic salts used in various combinations in most antacids: magnesium, aluminum, and calcium. Magnesium- and aluminum-based antacids (such as Di-Gel, Maalox, and Mylanta) use magnesium hydroxide and aluminum hydroxide, respectively, and are considered by some to be the most cost-effective heartburn drugs. A major side effect of magnesium hydroxide is diarrhea, while the most common side effect of aluminum hydroxide is constipation. Both can also interfere with calcium intake.

Antacids high in calcium—Tums, Rolaids, Titralac, and Alka-2—are probably the strongest, but they, too, can be constipating if too much is consumed. Calcium carbonate products, used for centuries in the form of chalk powder and oyster shell, are probably the most powerful antacids. Such antacids should not be used by people who have kidney disease, because there have been rare cases of hypercalcemia (elevated levels of calcium in the blood) found in people taking calcium carbonate for long periods. This can lead to kidney failure. Only calcium-containing antacids have this potential side effect, however.

When choosing an antacid, reflux sufferers ought to know that the peppermint used to flavor many of these tablets works as an LES relaxant and may be counterproductive. In any case, tablets must be chewed thoroughly in order to be effective.

Sodium bicarbonate, or baking soda, is the active ingredient in many of the seltzer antacids on the market, such as Alka-Seltzer and Bromo-Seltzer. It is less powerful than the other types of antacids on the market. Users of seltzer antacids must beware, because these medications when combined with stomach acid can produce large amounts of gas that can escape in the form of powerful burps. These antacids also should not be used by people on low-salt diets or by those with high blood pressure, heart disease, diabetes, glaucoma, or a history of stroke, because one Alka-Seltzer tablet, for example, contains 311 milligrams of sodium, more than half the amount needed by a healthy adult. At some fine restaurants, particularly in Europe, a bottle of mineral water is placed on the table. These mineral waters contain up to 5 grams of bicarbonate per quart and work to neutralize acid.

Because no single agent is perfect, many antacids combine several ingredients that are designed to balance out one another's side effects. Maalox, for example, combines magnesium hydroxide and aluminum hydroxide. One popular over-the-counter medication for heartburn, Gaviscon, combines antacids with alginic acid, a substance derived from marine algae. Its unique action creates a "raft" that floats on the gastric sea and helps block reflux.

Many doctors recommend taking commercial antacids both one hour and three hours after meals and at bedtime. The usual recommended dosage is one to two tablespoons or tablets each time.

## Histamine $H_2$-Receptor Antagonists

For chronic reflux, doctors may prescribe medications to reduce acid in the stomach. A long-accepted treatment for peptic ulcers, histamine $H_2$-receptor antagonists—or $H_2$ blockers—are now often used as well when GERD symptoms or esophagitis don't respond to antacids or changes in eating habits.

$H_2$ blockers work by blocking the effect of histamine, which stimulates gastric acid, and thereby decreasing the amount of acid produced by the stomach. They act directly on the stomach's acid-secreting cells to stop them from making hydrochloric acid, particularly during the night when acid gathers in the stomach and can wash back into the esophagus. $H_2$ blockers are generally more effective than antacids, but they are still not perfect. Studies show they completely heal only about 60 percent of cases of esophagitis, for example, and are even less effective against severe cases.

Cimetidine, the first $H_2$ blocker on the market (sold as Tagamet), was considered a major breakthrough in gastrointestinal drug therapy. In fact, its discoverer, Sir James Black, won the 1988 Nobel Prize for medicine on the strength of this development. Other $H_2$ blockers available in the United States include ranitidine (Zantac), famotidine (Pepcid), and nizatidine (Axid).

All four $H_2$ blockers are available by prescription as well as in lower dosages over the counter, as liquids, tablets, or capsules. If heartburn is troublesome only at night, a single dose taken in the evening may be sufficient; more frequent treatments are needed if symptoms occur throughout the day and night. Each of these four $H_2$ blockers are equally effective, so switching to another when one fails to work is likely to be fruitless. Increasing the dose, however, may be helpful.

$H_2$ blockers can occasionally have mild side effects, such as headache, dizziness, anxiety, sleeplessness, and depression. Cimetidine, moreover, is weakly anti-androgenic and may have feminizing effects such as breast development or loss of sex drive, in men. These are very rare, though, and, in any case, are reversible when the drug is stopped. Also, patients should avoid alcohol when using $H_2$ blockers, as they may produce a higher blood alcohol level.

While they are considered relatively safe, some doctors warn that self-treatment with these over-the-counter remedies may cause sufferers to mistake serious conditions for heartburn, delaying diagnosis and proper treatment.

## Prokinetic Agents

Prokinetics, or gastrokinetics as they are occasionally called, are a wide-ranging group of drugs that increase the speed at which the stomach empties of food, acid, and fluids. They also may strengthen esophageal peristalsis and improve LES tone. Usually used instead of or in addition to $H_2$ blockers, they are reserved for severe cases of GERD only.

Cisapride (Propulsid), the newest of these agents, was pulled from the American market in 2000 after it was linked to more than three hundred reports of heart-rhythm abnormalities, including more than eighty deaths. Its predecessors, bethanechol (Urecholine) and metoclopramide (Reglan), are still available by prescription. Side effects of bethanechol—which, in general, is no longer used—include increased salivation and gastric production, cramping, blurred vision, and frequent urination. Metoclopramide can produce muscle spasms, restlessness, and drowsiness. Both of them can interfere with the absorption of other drugs.

## Proton-Pump Inhibitors

Proton-pump inhibitors, or blockers, are the newest class of anti-GERD drugs and are much more effective than $H_2$ blockers at lowering the production of gastric acid and the amount of gastric secretions.

The proton-pump inhibitors—also known as acid-pump inhibitors—suppress acid secretion in the stomach by inactivating a specific enzyme responsible for the final step of acid release in the stomach. Available only by prescription for now, these medications have been like magic bullets for many patients with severe GERD. Omeprazole (Prilosec), lansoprazole (Prevacid), rabeprazole (Aciphex), pantoprazole (Protonix), and esomeprazole (Nexium) can reduce gastric-acid secretion by more than 95 percent without causing systemic side effects.

These medications are the drugs of choice for erosive esophagitis, although this condition usually recurs when the drug is stopped. Omeprazole, which like all the proton-pump inhibitors is impressive in its ability to heal esophagitis and alleviate heartburn, is the only one with FDA approval for repeated courses of treatment for erosive esophagitis.

Such effectiveness does not come without cautions, however. Animal studies have shown that prolonged use of these drugs can be associated with the growth of stomach tumors. Such tumors have not occurred in humans, though, after more than fifteen years of use. The drugs are also expensive and may cause the gastrointestinal tract to be more susceptible to bacterial infections.

Still, despite these concerns, proton-pump inhibitors have found a firm place in the treatment of reflux esophagitis and of patients with unremitting respiratory symptoms of GERD.

## Other Drugs
Another drug, sucralfate (Carafate), developed in Japan to treat ulcers, has also been used to relieve gastroesophageal reflux. It works by forming a protective coating over the stomach lining, but it is difficult to administer, is poorly absorbed, causes constipation, and may interfere with other drugs being taken. As a result, it is seen as no match for the $H_2$ blockers or proton-pump inhibitors.

## Combination Therapies
Several studies have looked at combining various anti-GERD drugs to enhance the effectiveness of each. One

study has suggested, for instance, that a combination of over-the-counter antacids and $H_2$ blockers may be the best remedy for those who experience heartburn after meals. Both types of drugs work to relieve GERD but have different timing mechanisms. Antacids neutralize acid already in the stomach and work quickly, but the effect lasts only an hour or two. $H_2$ blockers, meanwhile, suppress acid production, which itself takes from sixty to ninety minutes to begin—but their benefits continue for nine to twelve hours.

For more severe cases of reflux, some doctors prescribe a combination of $H_2$ blockers or proton-pump inhibitors with prokinetic drugs.

### Herbal Remedies
A number of herbs and other natural remedies have proven helpful in the treatment of symptoms of heartburn.

Chamomile is known for its soothing effects on the digestive tract. A cup of bagged chamomile tea, or two or three teaspoons of dried chamomile flowers in a cup of boiling water, is a surefire way to help the problem, some sufferers say.

Ginger, another well-known digestive herb, has been a folk remedy for heartburn for centuries. James Duke, author of *The Green Pharmacy*, recommends one teaspoon of freshly grated ginger root per cup of boiling water. Steep for ten minutes and drain before drinking.

Licorice has been proven effective in several studies. In one, researchers gave heartburn sufferers either antacids alone or antacids plus a licorice extract. Those who got the licorice reported experiencing more relief. Licorice is said to increase the mucus coating of the esophageal lining, helping it resist the irritating effects of stomach acid. Deglycyrrhizinated licorice, or DGL, is available in pill or liquid form. It is safe to take indefinitely.

Catnip, papaya tea, marshmallow root, and fennel have

all been said to aid in digestion and act as a buffers to stop heartburn. Eating fresh papaya or pineapple is also known to be an effective digestive aid. Many Chinese restaurants, for example, serve pineapple in slices or chunks following a meal.

On the less appealing end, some people swear by raw potato juice, three times a day, to alleviate heartburn. And a homeopathic remedy with the unappetizing name of vomit nut, or nux vomica, is also touted by naturopathic followers as a heartburn fix. It is made from the seeds of the *Strychnos nux-vomica* tree, which contain small amounts of strychnine. Strychnine acts as a bitter, increasing the flow of gastric juice.

Anyone who wishes to treat reflux using these medications should know that herbal remedies do not undergo safety testing and are not FDA approved. Note also that toxic reactions have been associated with some herbal remedies, though not necessarily those discussed here.


## Surgical Options

Ninety-five percent of GERD cases are controlled successfully through medication, but for a few patients—and only a few patients—surgery is the best option. Surgery may be preferable, for example, for young patients for whom the prospect of lifelong proton-pump treatment is unappealing. Other likely candidates for surgery are people with erosive esophagitis that does not improve with drug therapy, strictures that recur despite treatment, or pneumonia or recurrent, reflux-induced respiratory problems that don't improve with drug therapy.

The goal of GERD surgery is to tighten the LES. Fundoplication, the most common operation for GERD, is generally effective and can reduce or eliminate the need for GERD medications in most patients. Meanwhile, radiofrequency ablation and the Bard Endoscopic Suturing System are still in the trial stages but show encouraging results.

*Fundoplication* The most common antireflux operation is the Nissen (360-degree) fundoplication. Also known as a stomach wrap, the operation creates a vacuum effect that prevents stomach acid from surging upward.

This procedure involves literally grabbing a portion of the top of the stomach and looping it around the lower end of the esophagus and LES to create an artificial sphincter, or pinch valve. It prevents the reflux of acid from the stomach back up into the esophagus (*see* Figure 2.3). The wrap must be tight enough to prevent the acid from coming back up but not so tight that food can't enter the stomach and a satisfying belch can't escape.

After undergoing fundoplication, about 90 percent of patients are free of heartburn. Fundoplication also cures GERD-induced asthmatic or respiratory symptoms in about 85 percent of patients. In addition, fundoplication improves abnormal peristalsis in about half of the patients and it may also enhance stomach emptying.

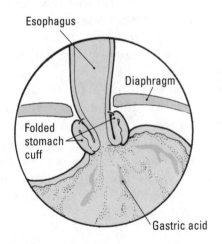

**FIGURE 2.3: GASTROESOPHAGEAL REFLUX SURGERY**

In a procedure called fundoplication, which is used to treat GERD, a surgeon folds the top of the stomach around itself to create a high-pressure zone that functions as a lower esophageal sphincter.

Increasingly, surgeons are performing fundoplication as a laparoscopic procedure, which means that it is done with special instruments and cameras that are inserted into tiny incisions in the upper abdomen. Patients recover faster after this than they would if a large surgical cut was needed. Most patients go home within two days of the surgery and within a week or two are able to swallow without pain or the feeling that food is catching on the way down.

Many experts now believe that because of the ease of laparoscopy, surgery should be considered as primary treatment for patients who normally would be candidates for long-term drug therapy. One study reported that the cost of surgery is less than a lifetime of treatment with proton-pump inhibitors.

Still, complications can occur even with minimally invasive surgeries, and patients should always consider any elective operation very carefully. Possible complications of fundoplication include bowel obstruction and injury to nearby organs—and the surgery may need to be repeated if the wrap slips or is too loose. The laparoscopic procedure is more difficult in certain patients, including those who are obese, have a short esophagus, or have had previous surgery in the abdominal area.

There are several variations of the fundoplication procedure. One finding favor with some surgeons uses only a partial wrap. This procedure may also involve repair of a hiatal hernia, if present, which involves taking the segment of the stomach that has protruded above the diaphragm and putting it back where it belongs. Once one of the most commonly performed operations, hiatal hernia repair on its own is now seldom done.

## Radiofrequency Ablation
The FDA recently approved tests of a procedure that uses radiofrequency energy to treat GERD. The procedure in-

volves applying controlled radiofrequency energy through a flexible catheter run down through the lower esophageal sphincter muscle. It takes under an hour and helps the valve stop reflux.

Known as the Stretta procedure, the technique "zaps" the LES and upper part of the stomach with radio-frequency energy, causing the lining of the lower esophagus to expand slightly. As a result, the valve tightens up, creating a more effective barrier between the esophagus and the stomach.

Results of a six-month follow-up study found that 70 percent of those who underwent this minimally invasive procedure were able to stop taking all GERD medications. However, complications such as esophageal perforation can occur, and long-term results are anxiously awaited.

Patients undergoing radiofrequency ablation can get back to their regular activities the next day.

## Bard Endoscopic Suturing System

Another new minimally invasive procedure in trials that has been shown to effectively treat GERD is the Bard Endoscopic Suturing System. The technique, which also recently won FDA approval, uses a thin, flexible endoscopic tube with something that resembles a miniature sewing machine at its tip. In a procedure that requires no incision or anesthesia, the device is inserted down the patient's throat and is used to place stitches on either side of the LES. The doctor then ties the sutures together to tighten the valve.

As with the Stretta procedure, patients go home the same day. After a six-month follow-up, 75 percent of patients no longer needed GERD medications.

# 3

# Functional Dyspepsia

*Dyspepsy is the ruin of most things: empires, expeditions,*
*and everything else.*
—Thomas de Quincey

You're having trouble with your stomach. It's not heart-burn, but it may be related to eating. You feel uncomfortable. You feel bloated and full. You complain of nausea and sometimes even vomit. Probably, you say you are suffering from indigestion.

Doctors call it dyspepsia. The literal translation of the word is "bad digestion." It is derived from the Greek *dys,* which means bad, and *peptein,* which means "to cook" or "to digest."

The term *functional dyspepsia* (FD) is used to describe chronic and persistent upper-abdominal pain that is often related to eating but not attributable to any identifiable cause, such as peptic ulcer disease. Peptic ulcer disease produces similar symptoms, and functional dyspepsia is in fact sometimes called non-ulcer dyspepsia.

In most cases, the uncomfortable upper-abdominal

symptoms seem to arise after eating, but there's no difficulty swallowing. Sometimes the discomfort appears during the meal, but more often it shows up about a half hour later. It tends to come and go in spurts.

The condition affects about one-quarter of the population—twice as many people as have peptic ulcer disease—and touches men and women equally. The problem is responsible for a significant percentage of visits to primary-care doctors.

Many people with functional dyspepsia suspect that they are suffering from ulcers, but later are found not to be. Dyspepsia has many possible causes, some of which are more easily diagnosed than others, but the cause of functional dyspepsia is not known. Even more frustrating is the fact that there is no surefire way to cure it.

## Is It an Ulcer?

"Do I have an ulcer?" It's the first question on most sufferers' minds, and not an unreasonable one, considering that 10 percent of Americans develop a peptic ulcer at some time in their lives. And it is important that the question of whether an ulcer exists be answered quickly, for while functional dyspepsia generally does not cause serious complications, an ulcer can. The ulcer can be treated with medications; FD in most cases does not respond well to medications.

Peptic ulcers are raw, craterlike breaks in the mucosal lining of the digestive tract. They occur in the stomach (these are gastric ulcers) or duodenum (duodenal ulcers) and are linked to the erosive action of gastric acid as well as sometimes to a reduction in protective mucus (*see* Figure 3.1). In essence, with an ulcer, the stomach, which is designed to digest foods, is digesting a part of its own lining. These localized, usually circular craters are rarely more than an inch in diameter.

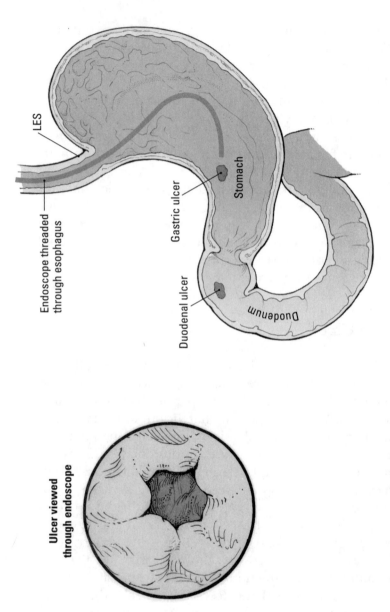

**Ulcer viewed through endoscope**

LES

Endoscope threaded through esophagus

Gastric ulcer

Stomach

Duodenal ulcer

Duodenum

## FIGURE 3.1: PEPTIC ULCERS

Peptic ulcers are raw, craterlike breaks in the mucosal lining of the stomach and duodenum. Physicians can use an endoscope to view the stomach and duodenum and confirm the presence of an ulcer.

Irritating substances, including aspirin and other non-steroidal anti-inflammatory drugs (NSAIDs) can cause ulcers. Tobacco is another cause; cigarette smoking has also repeatedly been shown to impair ulcer healing, although the reason is not clear. Stress is thought to play a role too, but the evidence now favors the theory that stress aggravates ulcers rather than causes them. Studies also show there is also a genetic component to the development of ulcers, as peptic ulcers sometimes run in families. They occur more often in people with type-O blood than in those with other blood types.

In the early 1980s, researchers made a major discovery with respect to peptic ulcers when they identified *Helicobacter pylori*, a spiral bacterium with an affinity for the stomach, as a major culprit in ulcer disease *(see* box, The Germ of Discovery, and Figure 3.2). Some say this organism is the cause of most peptic ulcers, or at least most of those not caused by NSAIDs, and in fact, at least 90 percent of people with duodenal ulcers and 75 to 85 percent of those with gastric ulcers are infected with the organism. Evidently, *H. pylori* infection weakens the protective mucus coating of the stomach and duodenum, allowing acid to get through to the sensitive lining beneath. Both the acid and the bacteria irritate the lining and cause a sore, or ulcer *(see* Figure 3.2). *H. pylori* may also cause high levels of acid secretion by the stomach. *H. pylori* itself is able to survive in stomach acid because it secretes enzymes that neutralize the acid.

## THE GERM OF DISCOVERY

In 1982, Australian researchers Barry J. Marshall and J. Robin Warren identified a corkscrew-shaped organism, *Helicobactor pylori,* as a cause of gastritis and a major factor in peptic ulcer disease.

They discovered the *Helicobacter pylori* bacterium (formerly called *Campylobacter pylori* ) residing below the mucus layer and on the surface

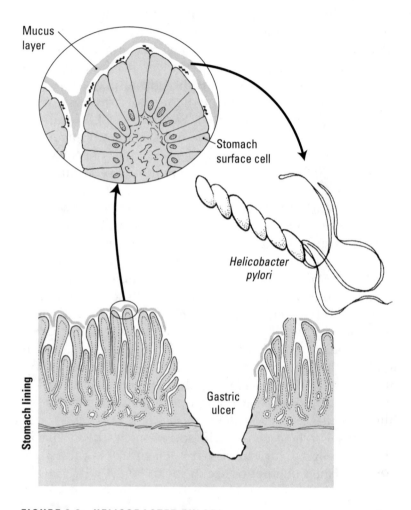

**FIGURE 3.2: *HELICOBACTER PYLORI***

*Helicobacter pylori* thrives in the stomach because it can produce large quantities of urease, an enzyme that generates ammonia, to neutralize the acid that quickly kills other bacteria. The corkscrew-shaped *H. pylori* attaches itself to the surface of stomach cells after twisting through the mucus that protects the lining from corrosive gastric juices. Scientists believe that *H. pylori* contributes to ulcers in several ways, including thinning the protective mucus layer, poisoning nearby cells with ammonia or other toxins, or even increasing gastric acid production.

lining, or epithelium, of the stomach. Since then, *H. pylori* has been confirmed as a key factor in peptic ulcer disease and a primary cause of gastritis.

What is fascinating about *H. pylori* is its prevalence. More than half of the world's population is infected with the bacterium, yet most people exhibit no symptoms. The infection becomes more common with age, too; in the United States, 50 percent of the population harbor the organism by age fifty-five. Researchers believe that *H. pylori* is probably transmitted through personal contact, especially in crowded living facilities.

Nearly all individuals with duodenal ulcers and at least three-fourths of those with gastric ulcers are infected with *H. pylori*. However, the strongest evidence of *H. pylori*'s causal relationship with peptic ulcer is that eradicating the bug nearly completely eliminates ulcer recurrence. Certain types of gastric lymphomas (malignant tumors of the lymphoid system) and gastric cancers have also been linked to *H. pylori*, and antibiotic treatment has resulted in the regression of some of the lymphomas.

---

A number of tests may be employed to confirm the presence of *H. pylori*, which then can be treated with various combinations of antibiotics and proton-pump inhibitors or other drugs.

The final chapter on *H. pylori* and its link to ulcers, however, is still being written. *H. pylori* is probably the world's most common infection, affecting more than half of all humans, particularly those over age fifty-five. Yet only 15 to 20 percent of people who harbor *H. pylori* will ever develop an ulcer. Why, then, do all who are infected not have ulcers?

Clearly, there is more to learn about *H. pylori* and its role in the development of peptic ulcers. In the meantime, there are many patients with dyspepsia, even without ulcers, who are being treated as if *H. pylori* were the cause of their stomach maladies. At the same time, the incidence of peptic ulcers is falling. Most likely, development of ulcers depends on the characteristics of the infected person, specific features of the *H. pylori* present, and other factors not yet discovered.

## Diagnosing Functional Dyspepsia

As far as symptoms go, functional dyspepsia and ulcer disease have far more similarities than differences. Dyspepsia may occur in patients with or without ulcers. Both have a chronic history, and both seem to be stress-related and affect people of all ages. In many cases, symptoms of each condition respond to treatment with placebo. And with each condition, palpating the patients' abdomen may elicit tenderness.

In order to properly diagnose FD, ulcer disease, or both, and prescribe treatment, your doctor will want to take a complete history and get complete details about the frequency of pain, how long it has persisted, and when it is most severe. Discomfort that is worse on an empty stomach and is relieved by eating suggests a duodenal ulcer, but that by itself isn't definitive. Questions will also address health habits, such as smoking and alcohol consumption, as well as the condition's effect on sleep: pain that often awakens a person during the night points to ulcer disease, as does whether that person gains any relief from antacids or $H_2$ blockers taken at bedtime. The physician will also want to know whether other family members have ever been diagnosed with a peptic ulcer.

Symptoms that may point to an ulcer include the following:

☞ Evidence of bleeding, such as vomiting blood or material that resembles coffee grounds, or passing black stools
☞ Repeatedly vomiting large amounts of sour liquid and food, which can signal an obstructing ulcer

☞ Sudden, overwhelming pain, a rare but frightening signal that the ulcer has perforated the stomach or duodenal wall.

Pain is the most common symptom of an ulcer. The pain usually is a dull, gnawing ache that comes and goes for several days or a week at a time. It also frequently occurs two or three hours after a meal, or in the middle of the night, and is relieved by food.

To determine whether symptoms are caused by an ulcer, the doctor may order an endoscopy or an upper gastrointestinal (GI) series, which is an X-ray examination of the esophagus and stomach using barium as the contrast medium: the patient drinks a chalky liquid containing barium, after which the radiologist takes a series of X rays as the barium flows through the esophagus and stomach. Some doctors may be wary of ordering expensive tests, however, because insurers or managed-care plans may balk at paying and because the results are unlikely to influence initial treatment strategies.

Diagnosis of functional dyspepsia is further complicated by the disorder's resemblance to other illnesses besides ulcers. Gastritis, gastroesophageal reflux, irritable bowel syndrome, chronic pancreatitis (inflammation of the pancreas), stomach cancer, and hepatobiliary pain (pain originating from the liver or gall bladder) can all cause similar symptoms to those of FD (*see* box, Functional Dyspepsia: What Else Could It Be?) In short, a clinical examination may not be enough to exclude an ulcer or other disease that may be causing a patient's symptoms.

As a first treatment step, a doctor will likely prescribe one or more drugs that curtail acid secretion to see if the dyspepsia clears up or will order a blood test for *H. pylori*. If the blood test is positive, antibiotics to eradicate the bug will be prescribed. If symptoms do not improve after a few weeks, the next step probably will be endoscopy to check for ulcers.

Patients over forty-five with a new onset of dyspepsia or

## FUNCTIONAL DYSPEPSIA: WHAT ELSE COULD IT BE?

At least some of the distress associated with functional dyspepsia (FD) is due to the nagging fear that a more serious condition may be going undetected. Although this is hardly ever the case, especially when symptoms persist for months or years without worsening, even the suggestion of a serious problem is troubling. Fortunately, more serious ailments have characteristics that set them apart from FD.

☛ **Gallstones** (*see* Figure 3.3) Stones can dwell silently in the gallbladder or can produce painful attacks, typically after a large, high-fat dinner. The pain is usually located just under the right rib cage and may radiate to the right shoulder or back.

If a stone becomes impacted in the "neck" of the gallbladder (near the cystic duct that drains into the bile duct) and inflames the gallbladder, the patient may experience extreme tenderness when a hand is pressed below the ribs on the right side. He or she may develop fever and an elevated white-blood-cell count. Jaundice (a yellowing of the skin and the whites of the eyes), dark urine, and pale stools occur when a gallstone slips out of the gallbladder and obstructs the duct that drains bile from the liver into the duodenum. Symptomatic gallstones are usually treated surgically (by laparoscopy). In some cases, gallstones may be dissolved by the use of oral bile salts or crushed by use of a procedure that uses shock waves.

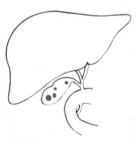

**FIGURE 3.3: GALLSTONES**

☞ **Stomach cancer** (*see* Figure 3.4) Malignancies of the stomach generally occur later in life, after age fifty. Tumors that burrow into the stomach wall often produce symptoms that resemble those associated with ulcers. Eating a full meal can become impossible if growths extrude into the hollow of the organ or spread through the stomach wall, making it too stiff to expand. Warning signs include bleeding, persistent vomiting, a constant sense of nausea or fullness that interferes with normal eating, and weight loss. Stomach cancer usually requires the surgical removal of all or part of the stomach.

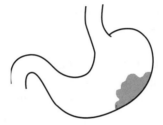

**FIGURE 3.4: STOMACH CANCER**

those whose dyspepsia is associated with additional worrisome symptoms such as weight loss, dysphagia (difficulty in swallowing), gastrointestinal bleeding, or anemia (low red-blood-cell count) should be evaluated promptly for underlying malignancies. Only after tests and drug trials fail to pinpoint another cause is the condition labeled FD.

Once diagnosed, FD is sometimes classified into types: ulcer-like dyspepsia, in which the main symptom is pain; motility-like dyspepsia, in which the primary symptoms may be bloating, fullness, and gas distension of the abdomen; and reflux-like dyspepsia, in which heartburn is the main symptom. These subgroups are not considered important from a clinical point of view, however, because there is a significant overlap among them and because many patients can't be classified.

## Causes of Functional Dyspepsia

Although there are several theories, we really don't know what causes the symptoms of FD. Many experts don't think that excess gastric acid is to blame, as studies have found no irregularities in acid secretion among dyspeptic patients and no correlation between symptoms and increased acid production. Still, the theory remains under consideration, as does one suggesting that abdominal pain associated with FD is caused by acid leaking through mucosa that has been altered in some way. Some other ideas about FD's cause are as follows:

*Abnormal motility or sensation* It is possible that the symptoms of FD are due to abnormal motility, or spontaneous movement of the digestive tract. Several such defects have been identified in some patients with FD. Some patients' stomachs empty more slowly than normal, so food is retained for a longer period of time. Such patients feel as though food is not leaving the stomach; they fill up quickly during a meal and may belch or burp. A mechanical failure of gastric contractions to empty the stomach may be the problem here. In addition, some FD patients have been shown to have relatively stiff stomach walls, so that rather little distension can occur after a meal. Other studies have shown that some people with FD have heightened gut sensations. Balloons inflated in the stomachs of patients with FD cause discomfort at volumes not perceived in healthy volunteers. Research and clinical studies are just now beginning to look at the complicated set of muscles and nerves and interactions responsible for moving the contents of the stomach.

*H. pylori infection* The role of *H. pylori* infection in FD is highly controversial. While the bacterium is an established cause of both gastritis and ulcers, its relationship to FD is much less convincing. *H. pylori* infection is only slightly more common in people with FD than it is in the general population, and although it may be that the organism contributes to FD symptoms in some cases, there is currently no way to distinguish these people from those in whom the *H. pylori* is not the cause of FD. Moreover, eradicating *H. pylori* with antibiotics usually does not significantly improve FD symptoms. *H. pylori* is present in up to 50 percent of people, with its frequency increasing with a person's age. To date, studies have not clearly implicated the organism in dyspepsia.

*Duodenitis* Another condition that might produce symptoms of FD is duodenitis, a chronic inflammation of the lining of the duodenum. However, fewer than a fifth of FD sufferers have this condition. Most physicians regard duodenitis as an early precursor of peptic ulcer disease and treat it as they would an ulcer.

*Psychological factors* Although scientific data are scarce, it seems that emotions can play an important role in the development of some cases of dyspepsia. We know that psychological factors can produce responses in the gut, but we're still trying to pinpoint the mind's exact influence in dyspepsia. One study focused on a man with a gunshot-induced fistula, or opening in the abdominal wall, that allowed his stomach to be observed, and found that when the man experienced fear, anger, or impatience, his stomach mucosa became pale and produced smaller quantities of gastric juices than normal. Another study demonstrated that gastric acid secretions increased in young men while they were reading erotic literature. However, it is not clear how these changes might cause dyspepsia.

*Diet* "Dyspepsia is more often the effect of overeating and overdrinking than any other cause," observed William Beaumont, a pioneer in the study of the digestive process, in 1833. Indeed, individuals with dyspepsia often attribute their symptoms to their diets. Overeating, certainly, can result in dyspeptic symptoms—we all know what it feels like after gorging on a holiday meal, for example; never again, we vow. One of the problems in such circumstances is that the stomach sends a signal to the brain that it is full, but the message takes twenty minutes to get there. A holiday reveler can stuff in a couple of pieces of pumpkin pie, with ice cream, quite easily during that waiting period. Additionally, certain fatty foods and fatty acids that delay gastric emptying are often blamed for dyspepsia, even if we don't eat too much. This connection makes sense because fat ingestion not only delays gastric emptying but also increases distension of the stomach. However, in one study, when people with a professed sensitivity to fats ate high-fat foods that were disguised, they did not experience dyspepsia. Substances like alcohol and coffee may also aggravate symptoms.

*Drugs* Nonsteroidal anti-inflammatory agents, especially aspirin, can cause dyspepsia, ulcers, and gastritis. A number of other drugs, such as opiates, iron preparations, and digitalis, may also cause dyspepsia, although how they do so is not yet known.

## Treating Functional Dyspepsia

The good news about functional dyspepsia is that it will not kill you. The bad news is that there isn't much that modern medicine has to offer by way of a cure.

Many patients are initially thankful when they get their diagnosis of functional dyspepsia—at least it isn't an ulcer or, worse, a malignancy. But the sense of relief can soon fade when they find out that they probably will have to continue living with the problem for the rest of their lives.

Were the problem an ulcer, at least they'd be cured with a short course of treatment with medications. With FD, however, no drug is really effective. Still, for some people, the knowledge that their condition isn't something more serious may cause the symptoms to disappear or at least become less important in the patient's life. For others, however, the symptoms will continue unchanged.

There is no scientific basis for a person with FD to choose one medication over another, because all of the potential choices seem to benefit only a minority of affected persons. In contrast to an ulcer, where there is a distinct pathological problem—a break in the stomach lining—for which there is specific medical treatment, with FD, the stomach and duodenal lining is intact, no pathological problem can be identified by X ray or endoscopy, and, normally, there is no excess gastric acid production or demonstrated motility problem—so drugs to correct these conditions are often unhelpful. Moreover, many clinical studies show that patients respond no better to drugs than to placebos. Nevertheless, doctors often prescribe treatment because the drugs are safe and, in fact, can have placebo effects for some patients. (Actually, in almost all clinical trials, from 25 to 60 percent of patients respond to placebo.)

In most cases, antacids are the preferred placebo. They are safe and quite inexpensive, and the side effects are few. $H_2$ blockers or proton-pump inhibitors are sometimes given, usually for short-term treatment. The prokinetic agent cisapride (Propulsid) has sometimes been used, particularly for the subgroup of patients who are bothered by nausea, fullness, and bloating, in the hope that those symptoms may be relieved by the drug's ability to speed up gastric emptying. The drug was pulled from the U.S. market in 2000, though, after it was linked to reports of heart-rhythm disturbances and more than eighty deaths.

Other medications are used as well. Like cisapride, the antibiotic erythromycin also encourages the stomach to empty and can be used instead of cisapride. Anticholinergics, medications that decrease contractions in the gastro-intestinal tract, such as hyoscyamine, may also be used for up to four to six weeks. Simethicone, a surfactant that rids the gut of gas bubbles, is safe and may serve as a placebo for the patient who complains of dyspepsia and flatulance.

Whether to treat an *H. pylori* infection, if present, in a person with FD is another consideration. There is no question that treatment of the bacteria is important in curing ulcers; studies show a remarkable decrease in ulcer recurrences when the organism is eradicated. But one cannot expect the same for FD symptom relief: A report in the *New England Journal of Medicine (NEJM)* showed that one year after successful antibiotic eradication of *H. pylori,* only 21 percent of FD patients were improved, compared to 7 percent who got a placebo. Another study published in the same *NEJM* issue could detect no significant difference in symptoms between patients treated with antibiotics or a placebo. Still, some doctors do try a course of antimicrobial therapy in patients who harbor *H. pylori* but have not responded to any other treatments. In any case, eradicating *H. pylori* has the added benefit of preventing a future risk of ulcers or gastric cancer.

## Living with Functional Dyspepsia

Live with it. In the end, that's what patients diagnosed with FD are going to have to do. Because the disorder is mysterious and difficult to treat, patients have to adapt their lives to accommodate their discomfort, whenever it happens and using whatever measures they can find to get relief.

As with reflux and other functional problems, FD requires using common sense. In essence, symptoms of FD may be improved by adopting a more healthful lifestyle. Inadequate diet, stress, fatigue, and inactivity all can aggravate the symptoms of FD. The following lifestyle modifications may prove helpful in relieving symptoms.

## Diet

☞ Avoid foods that trigger symptoms *(see* box, Foods and Drugs That May Aggravate Functional Dyspepsia, page 70)

☞ Stay away from large meals and overeating

☞ Eat smaller meals more often

☞ Chew your food slowly and completely

☞ Don't drink any beverages during meals, particularly if you feel full early on during a meal

☞ Keep away from activities that result in swallowing excess air, such as smoking, eating quickly, chewing gum, sipping through straws, and drinking carbonated beverages

☞ Don't lie down for at least two hours after eating

☞ Keep your weight under control

☞ Try herbal remedies such as ginger, aloe vera juice, ground anise seeds, and parsley in warm water to relieve indigestion. A new product, Gastro Ease, is being promoted as a natural formula to relieve FD based on traditional Chinese herbal medicine. It contains herbs such as ginger, licorice, and citrus rind and is said to treat the underlying causes of indigestion by working with the flow of energy in the body ("chi") to assist in the movement of digestion.

## Stress

☞ Pinpoint what is causing you stress and learn how to manage it. Biofeedback, stress management, exercise, or listening to soothing music may help.

☞ Relaxation techniques such as meditation, relaxed breathing, or guided imagery may prove useful.

## Fatigue

☞ Get enough rest

☞ Adopt a bedtime routine—go to bed and get up at the same time each day

☞ Don't sleep too much: be sure to keep your nighttime schedule and try to avoid naps

☛ Avoid caffeine after noon
☛ Exercise before seven P.M.

## Exercise
☛ Aerobic exercise three to five times a week for twenty to forty minutes each session is recommended, but make sure to get your doctor's permission before starting any new workout routine
☛ Start all exercise with a three- to five-minute warmup period
☛ Wait at least thirty minutes after eating before starting to exercise

---

### FOODS AND DRUGS THAT MAY AGGRAVATE FUNCTIONAL DYSPEPSIA

| | |
|---|---|
| Alcohol | Orange juice |
| Aspirin | Peanuts |
| Beans | Peppers |
| Caffeinated tea | Radishes |
| Coffee | Spicy sauces |
| Colas | Tobacco |
| Dairy products | Tomato juice |
| Fried foods | |
| Ibuprofen and other nonsteroidal anti-inflammatory drugs (NSAIDs) | |

---

# 4

# Irritable Bowel Syndrome

*Man should strive to have his intestines relaxed all the days of his life.*
—Moses Maimonides

Another common disorder of the intestines is irritable bowel syndrome (IBS). Its myriad of unpleasant symptoms affect tens of millions and have no known cause nor effective remedy.

Irritable bowel syndrome is probably the number-one reason why people see gastroenterologists, accounting for as many as 3.5 million physician visits and 2.2 million prescriptions per year. It accounts for an estimated 28 percent of patients seen by gastroenterologists and up to 12 percent of patients seen in primary-care offices.

The cost of all of this in dollars and cents is staggering. Studies have estimated the toll for caring for IBS patients at more than $8 billion in the United States alone. A Seattle study pegged the cost of caring for IBS sufferers at $4,044 per patient during the year in which they were diagnosed, a figure that is 35 percent higher than the average spent on treatment of patients with other illnesses.

For patients and doctors alike, irritable bowel syndrome is probably the most challenging of all functional gastrointestinal (GI) disorders. A recent study found that patients with IBS have a significantly lower quality of life than persons without the syndrome and that the illness is seriously underdiagnosed. In fact, only 4 percent of study participants who met the criteria for having IBS had been diagnosed with the condition by a physician.

Medical historians credit John Howship, of St. George's Infirmary in London, with providing the first scientific description of IBS, in an 1830 article entitled "Spasmodic Stricture of the Colon as an Occasional Cause of Confinement of the Bowels." His theory was that the abdominal pain and altered bowel habits of IBS sufferers stem from colonic dysmotility or spasm of the colon. Through the years, the condition has been called by many names—spastic colon, spastic bowel, colitis, mucous colitis, and functional bowel disease among them. None of these is quite accurate, however, hence the catchall term *irritable bowel syndrome.*

Today, IBS affects 10 to 22 percent of otherwise healthy adults. While it is thought to affect both sexes nearly equally, men and women may actually suffer from different symptoms. In any case, women are three to five times more likely to see a doctor for the problem than are men.

About 70 percent of patients who see physicians for IBS are considered to have "mild" symptoms, and their lives are minimally impacted. About 25 percent are said to have "moderate" symptoms, which may cause them to miss work occasionally. And roughly 5 percent of patients suffer from "severe" symptoms that considerably affect their daily lives. Symptoms usually begin in young adulthood, though they can occur in children as well.

The causes of irritable bowel syndrome are obscure. Many believe it stems from an abnormality in the contractions of the muscles of the colon, which can result from any of several factors, including distension or stretching, food residues, intestinal hormones, and stress. They may all combine to induce an abnormality in the rhythm of the bowels. On the other hand, some experts think the problem is primarily psychological in origin. Still others believe IBS to be a heightened sensitivity to stress. Whatever the cause, IBS remains quite real to the millions who suffer its symptoms.

Despite frustrating and sometimes debilitating symptoms that keep sufferers preoccupied with the toilet, most sufferers don't consult a doctor. There may be good reason not to; the cost of seeking out care may be high, and the drugs used to treat IBS not only are expensive, but also offer scarce evidence of effectiveness. And, in some cases, IBS patients are liable to undergo unnecessary surgeries. Many simply try to cope on their own, tolerating the symptoms or attempting to alleviate them by avoiding certain foods, taking over-the-counter remedies or herbal preparations, or trying stress-reduction techniques.

## What Is Irritable Bowel Syndrome?

Symptoms of irritable bowel syndrome usually begin to appear when a patient is anywhere between his or her twenties and forties. In a typical situation, you're a relatively healthy person, then one day you begin to suffer intermittent cramps in the lower abdomen. You have to move your bowels often, much more often than usual. And when you have to go, you have to get to a toilet right away.

Your stools are loose, watery, and possibly contain mucus—stuff you've never seen before in a bowel movement. Sometimes, you feel bloated and full of gas.

The cramps are relieved by a bowel movement (often diarrhea). After a while, however, the cramps return, but this time when you try to go to the bathroom, nothing happens. You're constipated.

Back and forth it goes: diarrhea, constipation, and pain and bloating in between.

You're probably suffering from irritable bowel syndrome, a catchall term for this mixed bag of symptoms, the most frequently reported of which is pain or discomfort in the abdomen, rather than a name for a solitary, specific complaint.

It's a common disorder with no known cause. People with IBS generally feel their pain subside after a bowel movement or passing gas. But they also may feel that they haven't fully emptied their rectum after a movement. While some patients may have daily episodes or continuous symptoms, others experience long symptom-free periods. These patterns may raise the question as to whether someone actually has irritable bowel syndrome as opposed to the occasional bowel complaints that may be considered part of the bowel's normal response to stress.

Sometimes, these bouts of bowel irregularities begin when one is about to undertake a stressful endeavor, such as taking a big exam or going out on a first date. "Nervous stomach" is what some would call it.

Whether it is IBS usually depends on frequency. The formal criterion for diagnosis is that symptoms have occurred during any three months of the previous twelve.

Fortunately, there is no organic basis for IBS. And doctors do not believe IBS is a forerunner of any more serious diseases, such as ulcerative colitis, Crohn's disease, or stomach cancer (*see* Chapter 5, Diseases with Symptoms Similar to Irritable Bowel Syndrome). But for the significant percentage of the population that experiences IBS, that's little comfort. They are suffering. If doctors can find nothing wrong, why are they suffering?

Doctors say that the irritable bowel is a disorder in the functioning of the intestinal tract. Some suspect disturbances in the functioning of nerves or muscles in the gut lay at the root; others believe abnormal processing of gut sensations in the brain may hold the key to at least some cases. Because no organic cause can be found, IBS often has been thought to be caused by emotional conflict, stress, or some other psychological factor. While such factors may worsen symptoms, however, researchers suggest that other factors are also at work.

## Motility and Transit

Because the spasmodic pain associated with IBS seems to emanate from the colon, numerous investigators have searched for the condition's cause in irregularities in the way food makes its way through this part of the gastrointestinal tract. Findings, however, have been inconsistent.

Colon motility (contractions of intestinal muscles and movement of its contents) is controlled by nerves, hormones, and electrical activity in the colon muscle. The electrical activity acts like a pacemaker and is similar to the mechanism that regulates heartbeat.

Movement of the colon propels the contents slowly back and forth, but mainly in the direction of the rectum. A few times a day, strong contractions move down the colon, pushing the contents ahead, resulting in a bowel movement.

Some researchers have found that the colon muscle of a person with IBS begins to spasm after only mild stimulation. The colon seems to be more sensitive and reactive than usual, they found, so it responds strongly to stimuli that would not affect other people. Sometimes, the spasms lead to diarrhea, other times to constipation. Other researchers, however, counter with studies showing that colonic motor activity is no different for IBS patients than for anyone else.

Some studies have suggested that diarrhea is associated with rapid small-intestinal transit and constipation with slow transit. In addition, there are studies that have shown that clustered contractions—short bursts of muscle activity separated by long rest periods—occur more often in the small intestines of IBS patients than other people and may be associated with abdominal pain. Still other studies, though, have found these contractions to be just as frequent in healthy people without symptoms. In short, studies have shown no consistent motility pattern in patients with IBS. While it appears that motility plays a role in IBS pain, that exact role remains a mystery.

## Perception

Another possible explanation for irritable bowel syndrome's bothersome symptoms is that people with IBS have a heightened awareness of the inner workings of their gut. In several well-known experiments in which balloons were inflated in the sigmoid colon, rectum, and small intestine, IBS patients usually had a much lower threshold for pain than healthy volunteers. Scientists believe that the lower threshold for internal pain may be related to the dispatch of nerve signals from the gut to the brain.

Indeed, people with IBS may just be more sensitive to a variety of ailments, perhaps their entire bodies are hyperreactive. People with irritable bowel complaints may also have more headaches, palpitations, chest tightness, shortness of breath, and chronic fatigue than the general population. They might feel pain more intensely, complain more about colds; some researchers even surmise that they suffer more anxiety and depression than other people and, when questioned, are more likely to regard themselves as being "sick."

## Hormone and Dietary Factors

Hormones produced in the GI tract, such as cholecystokinin, which stimulates gallbladder contractions after a meal, and motilin, which helps regulate bowel motility, have been suspected of triggering IBS symptoms, but studies have not been definitive. Researchers have also found that women with IBS may have more symptoms during their menstrual periods, suggesting that reproductive hormones can increase IBS symptoms.

Certain medicines—such as antacids, antibiotics, beta blockers, and narcotics—and foods may trigger spasms in some people. Sometimes the spasm delays the passage of stool, leading to constipation. Chocolate, dairy products, or large amounts of alcohol are frequent offenders in these cases. Some people simply can't tolerate certain dietary substances such as lactose (a sugar found in milk), fructose (a sugar found in fruit and used as a sweetener), and sorbitol (an artificial sweetener) and develop bloating and diarrhea as a result. In addition, though caffeine causes loose stools in many people, it is more likely to affect those with IBS.

Sometimes, bran may increase IBS symptoms. Wheat flour, too, is a culprit in some cases. On the other hand, some believe lack of fiber in the diet may contribute to IBS, but not everyone with IBS improves on a high-fiber diet. Some may even feel worse.

Fats can also contribute to IBS symptoms. Fat in any form (animal or vegetable) is a strong stimulant of colonic contractions after a meal. Many foods contain fat, especially meats, poultry skin, dairy products, vegetable oil, and margarine and shortening.

## Stress

Many experts are convinced that there is a strong psychological component to irritable bowel syndrome, and stress is known to stimulate colonic spasms in people with IBS. The process is not completely understood, but scientists point out that the colon is controlled partly by the nervous system. Some studies have shown significantly higher stress levels among people with IBS compared to healthy individuals. And stress reduction or relaxation training or counseling has helped to relax IBS symptoms in some people.

But even this theory is not ironclad, as there are many people—with and without IBS—who manifest gut reactions to stressful life events. The bad effects stress has on IBS may be no different from those it has upon any other disorder of the body.

## Psychological Factors

Despite the influence of emotions, there is no evidence that IBS is a completely imaginary complaint; the symptoms are real and troublesome enough in many cases to warrant attention. Yet there is one school of thought claiming that nearly all cases of IBS are psychological in nature, that the symptoms are merely the mind's attempt to take its focus off emotional problems that, if dwelled upon, could be even more upsetting to the person than the gastrointestinal distress. All of this remains in the theoretical realm, however.

It *is* a fact, though, that studies conducted at medical centers have found considerably more psychiatric problems among IBS patients than among healthy people or those with structural bowel diseases. Between 42 and 61 percent of patients with functional bowel disorders who are seen in gastrointestinal clinics also have a current psychiatric diagnosis—usually anxiety or depression, according to a report by Dr. Douglas A. Drossman of the University of North Carolina. But most patients do not see the psychiatric symptoms as being as important as their physical symptoms.

Despite this disturbing fact, many experts feel that formal psychiatric care is not needed for most IBS patients, nor has it proved especially helpful. On the other hand, some sessions with a good therapist may help patients manage their illness better. And such sessions could uncover and treat a problem with depression, for example, which may be either a cause or a result of the patient's IBS.

Psychiatric disorders frequently associated with severe IBS include trauma from childhood abuse, depression, anxiety, phobia, and somatization, a condition in which psychological stresses manifest as physical complaints. Sometimes, the onset of IBS symptoms is preceded by a life-threatening event or a major crisis such as a divorce or a loved one's death.

Although it is important to attend to the emotional problems of those suffering from IBS, it appears that a person's psychological state is not the only factor to be considered when trying to determine the origin of the irritable gut. That said, however, there is some evidence that antidepressants may be useful in treating IBS. The reasons are not clear why. It may be that when patients feel less depressed, they complain less about their bowels. Or it may prove that the drugs used to treat depression actually have additional beneficial effects on gut function.

Why some people with IBS go to the doctor and others don't is also a good question, though it appears that those who do seek care may be experiencing more discomfort. It may be that psychosocial factors influence this decision, too: attitudes toward illness and pain are important factors and may date back to behaviors learned in childhood. It appears that IBS sufferers are more prone to chronic illness behavior and that this behavior may be learned. *Chronic illness behavior* is a term describing the depression and discouragement that often accompany life with chronic illness, and it may include the inability to sleep, weight loss, undernourishment, or the inability to hold a job. Some doctors see such behaviors as an involuntary response to living with chronic illness, but others look upon chronic illness behavior as no more than patients "acting ill" in order to secure some secondary gain, such as the attention of a spouse or child.

## Diagnosing Irritable Bowel Syndrome

Since there are no tests for irritable bowel syndrome, the illness must be diagnosed entirely by the symptoms being experienced by the patient and a limited number of tests to exclude the likelihood of an organic disease. Fortunately, a positive diagnosis usually can be made on the first visit to a doctor.

The doctor must take a complete medical history that includes a careful description of symptoms. A physical exam and laboratory tests likely will also be done, and a stool sample will probably be tested for evidence of bleeding. In some cases, the doctor may also perform diagnostic procedures such as endoscopy (specifically sigmoidoscopy) and possibly take X rays to find out if there is any evidence of disease such as colitis, colon cancer, or inflammatory bowel disease.

At this stage as few costly, invasive tests as possible are used to determine whether a patient is suffering from a specific, identifiable "organic" condition or irritable bowel syndrome. To accomplish this, experts in the treatment of gastrointestinal illnesses have developed a specific set of criteria to identify people with irritable bowel syndrome. A person is strongly suspected to have the syndrome if he or she has experienced abdominal pain or discomfort on a continuous or recurring basis for a total time of at least three of the previous twelve months, along with two of the following three additional features:

☞ The abdominal pain or discomfort is relieved with a bowel movement
☞ The onset of the pain is associated with a change in the frequency of stool
☞ The onset of the pain is associated with a change in the consistency of stool

In addition, the following symptoms are not considered essential for diagnosis, but if present are considered support for the diagnosis. They may also be used to identify certain types of IBS.

☛ Abnormal stool frequency (more than three bowel movements per day or less than three per week)
☛ Abnormal stool form (unusually hard or loose stool more than one out of every four times)
☛ Abnormal stool passage (straining, urgency, or the feeling of incomplete evacuation more than one in four times)
☛ Passage of mucus more than once in every four defecations
☛ Bloating or the sensation of having a distended abdomen more than one out of every four days

In questioning the patient about symptoms and performing a clinical exam, the physician should assess the total picture, including the nature and timing of pain, bowel habits, and other complaints. IBS symptoms can vary widely; pain can range from mild to intense, but it rarely interferes with normal eating and usually does not awaken a person during the night.

An attempt should be made to correlate symptoms with specific foods and medications, with particular emphasis on the consumption of milk products (to rule out lactose intolerance) and foods and beverages that contain fructose or sorbitol. Patients may need to keep food diaries for a few weeks to see if they can identify foods that provoke symptoms.

At the same time, it is especially important to consider emotional and psychological triggers for a patient's symptoms. Physicians will want to know what prompted the visit and will want to ask about the patient's lifestyle and stress level. After all, it's not unusual for traumatic life events, such as divorce or the loss of a job, to wreak havoc on the bowels and psyche. The doctor must also try to establish that the patient has no serious mental disturbance. A referral to a mental-health professional may be indicated in some cases.

Doctors must also make sure to exclude the presence of organic diseases. To this end, they will ask questions about the pain being experienced:

☛ **To where does the pain radiate?** Pain caused by gallstones, for example, may radiate to the chest, while some ulcers may cause pain that radiates to the back. While patterns of pain for IBS are not so easily definable, the most frequently reported symptom is pain or discomfort in the abdomen that is poorly localized, migratory or variable in nature, and usually relieved by defecation.

☛ **Is the pain steady or cyclical?** Ulcer pain tends to be cyclical. It is relieved by eating but may come back in the middle of the night. By contrast, pain caused by cancer tends to be continuous.

☛ **Is there cramping?** Cramps may signal intestinal obstruction.

Other symptoms that accompany the pain may offer clues as to the cause of a patient's discomfort, too. If there is pain in the lower abdomen and a change in bowel movements, an abnormality in the large intestine may be present. A combination of pain and fever can signal inflammation (such as diverticulitis), which requires immediate medical attention.

Another major diagnostic clue is any bleeding in the digestive tract. People with IBS can have rectal bleeding, but it's usually due to trivial causes—internal hemorrhoids, for example—and never to IBS alone. Bright-red blood comes from the lower digestive tract, while black, tarry blood comes from the upper portion of the tract. If there is bleeding, more tests must be performed to determine the cause.

A physical exam will also be performed. During the

exam, the physician will look for tenderness in the abdomen. If it is located in the lower right part, it may signal appendicitis; in the upper right part, inflammation of the gallbladder or liver. The doctor will also check for masses caused by tumors, large cysts, or impacted stool.

A digital rectal exam is also usually part of the exam. In the exam, the doctor feels for masses in the rectum and, in males, the prostate. If a serious disorder is suspected, more tests will be ordered immediately.

Additional tests may include a complete blood count and erythrocyte sedimentation rate test, which measures the speed at which mature red blood cells settle; it can be used to screen for inflammatory disease. If the hemoglobin, white count, erythrocyte sedimentation rate, and temperature are normal and the patient's symptoms are typical of IBS, no further tests may be needed.

For patients with persistent diarrhea, stool samples will be examined for infectious agents that include intestinal parasites. Occasionally, the doctor may arrange for a three-day stool collection to check for excess fecal fat content (more than seven grams of fat per day) or weight (more than 200 grams of feces per day), neither of which is consistent with a diagnosis of IBS. Either may be an indicator instead of an organic problem such as inflammatory bowel disease, malabsorption, or even cancer.

And despite efforts to avoid expensive tests, a patient's age or atypical symptoms may persuade the doctor to conduct even more diagnostic procedures, such as sigmoidoscopy or colonoscopy.

A flexible sigmoidoscopy may be performed to check for tumors, particularly in people over the age of forty, or inflammatory bowel disease (*see* Chapter 5, Diseases with Symptoms Similar to Irritable Bowel Syndrome). The procedure, which permits observation of the rectum and sigmoid colon through a viewing tube and can be used to take a tissue sample, may be performed in the doctor's office with no anesthesia. Such a test, while somewhat uncomfortable, can also provide a measure of relief to the patient. In any patient over age forty, a colonoscopy or barium enema, may also be ordered to rule out colon cancer.

When it comes to tests, common sense should prevail: not every patient with a gut problem should get every test, especially because, unfortunately, no test can confirm IBS. Thus, patients should discuss each option carefully with the doctor before proceeding with any course of testing or treatment. Aggressive investigation may uncover an alternative diagnosis, or it may provide reassurance to patients and doctors that a potentially serious illness has not been overlooked.

The physical exam will usually not reveal anything other than perhaps a mildly tender abdomen in a patient with IBS. And lab tests are generally normal in IBS patients.

Despite the long list of possible tests, however, remember that an experienced gastroenterologist will likely be able to make a preliminary determination as to whether IBS is the problem on hearing the patient's initial story.

## Managing Irritable Bowel Syndrome

If you think that diagnosing IBS is tricky, wait until you try managing it. Diagnosis is only the beginning—the real quandary is figuring out a way to live with it.

While there may be comfort in knowing that the condition is benign, the relief probably won't last long because you'll soon find out that the prognosis for IBS sufferers can mean years—maybe a lifetime—of bowel distress.

If doctors knew what caused this group of symptoms, treatment would be easier and aimed at providing comfort and eliminating those causes. But that is not yet the case. As a result, treatment is directed at individual symptoms, and the process is somewhat hit-or-miss and complete relief is sometimes difficult to obtain. The frustration this can induce has sent many IBS sufferers into the world of alternative or complementary therapies to try such remedies as hypnosis, biofeedback, or herbs, with varying degrees of success.

Accordingly, the management of IBS requires a great deal of understanding between doctor and patient. When a patient has a clear-cut organic disease, such as an ulcer, the treatment plan is not a matter of debate. In contrast, the proper treatment of functional disorders such as irritable bowel syndrome is not so clear.

Patients need to educate themselves about IBS and receive adequate information from their physicians so they can learn to manage the syndrome and regain control over their lives. At least one study found that strong communication between doctor and patient reduced the number of IBS follow-up visits.

What is known about IBS is that something has disrupted the automatic functioning of the bowel, and the first task in management is to search for possible irritants coming from outside or arising from within the body. The natural place to start is with something consumed—foods, beverages, or drugs, for example.

Common sense should prevail in treating IBS, and so the first step should be the easiest: dietary measures. Patients should eliminate likely food triggers—caffeine, sorbitol-containing gum or beverages, dairy products, alcohol, apples and other raw fruits, fatty foods, and gas-producing vegetables like beans, cabbage, and broccoli—to see if symptoms subside. Some call it "eating bland." *(See* box, Foods That May Trigger Irritable Bowel Syndrome.)

## FOODS THAT MAY TRIGGER IRRITABLE BOWEL SYNDROME

| | |
|---|---|
| Apples and other raw fruits | Dairy products |
| Beans | Fatty foods |
| Broccoli | Margarine |
| Cabbage | Nuts |
| Caffeine | Orange and grapefruit juices |
| Cauliflower | Wheat products |
| Chewing gum, beverages, or | |
| foods sweetened with fructose | |
| or sorbitol | |

Should milk be found to be a problem, lactose-intolerant individuals can take supplements of the enzyme lactase if they can't always (or don't want to) avoid milk. There are also a host of lactose-free milk products on the market.

The most common dietary recommendation for IBS sufferers is adding fiber to increase the stool's bulk and speed the movement of contents through the gastrointestinal tract. The refined diet of the Western world, which is low in fiber, has been compared to the fiber-rich diets of much of the rest of the world, and our low fiber content has been blamed by some for the high rates of IBS in America. This connection, however, has not been proven, and a high-fiber diet does not always improve bowel symptoms. Still, many clinical trials have shown that bulking up on fiber does seem to relieve constipation and ease abdominal pain. It may even alleviate diarrhea.

To increase fiber intake, doctors usually recommend bran or a fiber supplement, such as psyllium or methylcellulose, available in many products found in supermarkets or drugstores. Fiber should be introduced gradually, however, because too much too soon can cause excessive gas, cramping, and bloating.

For some people, these dietary measures may be all that is needed to reduce symptoms and calm the belly. One study noted improvement in most patients who follow these recommendations, but many patients continue to have flare-ups after an initial response to therapy.

## When Problems Persist

There are certain occasions when doctors will consider the use of drug therapy for patients who continue to experience symptoms troublesome enough to impair daily function. While these drugs can't cure irritable bowel syndrome, they may help to ease symptoms.

To date, despite dozens of scientific trials, no drug has proven to be generally effective against IBS—yet data show that one-third to one-half of patients with functional complaints actually improve on placebo. In any case, there are times when the doctor may want to prescribe drugs for specific indications such as diarrhea, cramping, or pain.

*Anticholinergics* Drugs such as atropine and related agents, like dicyclomine (Bentyl), hyoscyamine (Levsin), and chlordiazepoxide (Librax), may relieve mild abdominal pain because as antispasmodics they reduce bowel spasms. People who often experience cramps after eating may obtain some relief if they take the antispasmodic medications before meals. The idea is to ensure maximum anticholinergic effect at the time symptoms are expected, while allowing minimum exposure to side effects.

*Antidepressants* Amitriptyline (Elavil) and desipramine (Norpramin) may sometimes be prescribed for patients who have diarrhea-predominant IBS. These tricyclic antidepressants should be used at low doses, however, and should be used only by patients who have diarrhea-predominant IBS, as they can cause constipation. The newer selective–seratonin-reuptake inhibitors (SSRIs), such as sertraline (Zoloft), may be helpful in treating abdominal pain in patients who suffer primarily from constipation-related IBS. Another SSRI, paroxetine (Paxil), may be used to treat abdominal pain in diarrhea-predominant IBS because of its anticholinergic antidiarrheal effect.

A Mayo Clinic study found that patients with gastrointestinal disorders taking antidepressants had no significant demonstrable changes in gastrointestinal motility. However, the patients did have a significant improvement in their gastrointestinal-symptom ratings and significant improvement in their overall sense of well-being.

Another study, from Belgium, looked at the effects of the SSRI citalopram on the physiology of the colon and found that when patients had balloons inflated in their colons, there was a slight relaxation of the colon. This was followed by an intravenous dose of citalopram. Patients reported a reduction of discomfort. The findings led the researchers to conclude that the drug may reduce visceral hypersensitivity by relaxing the colon.

Current research is focusing more on the gut-brain connection, which appears to play a role in IBS. Serotonin-like medications are among those being investigated. However, the first of these to be approved, alosetron (Lotronex), which works on the serotonin type III receptor, was a disaster and was pulled from the market just a year after winning FDA approval. The FDA urged Lotronex be taken off the shelves after receiving reports of three deaths and dozens of serious side effects in patients using the drug. In most of the reported cases, patients developed ischemic colitis, a potentially life-threatening inflammation of the large intestine that can occur when blood flow to that area of the gastrointestinal tract is blocked. In some cases, the drug caused constipation so severe that surgery was needed to unblock their intestines. One patient needed her colon removed.

Lotronex was the first new drug in decades for treatment of IBS and had been approved only for treatment of women whose main IBS problem was diarrhea.

*Loperamide (Imodium) and diphenoxylate (Lomotil)* These medications are generally recommended for patients whose main complaint is diarrhea. Loperamide, available over the counter, reduces the secretion of fluid by the intestine. Diphenoxylate, available by prescription only, helps to slow down intestinal contractions. It is related to codeine and contains atropine as well. Doctors generally favor preparations that don't contain codeine or other narcotics, because they may have adverse nervous-system effects, including sedation, drowsiness, and confusion.

## Beyond Drugs

Herbal remedies and other alternative or complementary therapies—as well as behavior techniques and psychotherapy—are being used frequently by patients with IBS when standard therapies don't work. One recent study conducted at the Royal London School of Medicine in England questioned 225 patients with intestinal problems. Of those with IBS, half were using complementary therapies. Most of these remedies are used to address the psychological components of the disorder.

Research shows that any of several stress-reducing techniques taught by psychologists or other specially trained medical professionals can help some patients. People should consider cost and availability in their community when choosing which ones to try, and should also know that there is little evidence available to prove the effectiveness of herbal remedies.

Among the most popular approaches are the following:

*Relaxation-response training and meditation* Simple and easy to learn, this technique helps reduce nervous-system activity and relaxes muscles. Meditation, including transcendental meditation (TM), has been shown to be very helpful in lowering blood pressure, for example. Similarly, the technique can help relax the intestinal muscle.

*Yoga* Some forms of yoga, the ancient Indian spiritual discipline that seeks to bring the body and mind into balance, have proven valuable to some IBS sufferers. Yoga, like meditation, can help the patient induce a form of self-relaxation. The ancient tradition, which emphasizes special breathing exercises, recognizes the intimate connection between the breath and the nervous system. The yogis believe that if one can learn to control the breath, he or she can learn to control, or at least influence, how he or she feels both emotionally and physically.

*Hypnosis* Hypnotherapy was strongly associated with improved IBS symptoms by one study presented in 2000 by researchers at the Eastern Virginia Medical School in Norfolk. About 85 percent of study participants who were given hypnosis sessions and audiotapes at home reported improvement in all IBS symptoms after fourteen weeks. Significant improvement was found in abdominal pain, bloating, stool consistency, and other involuntary body activities. After the course of hypnotherapy, the autonomic nervous system was less easily stimulated. The researchers theorized that the calming effect of hypnosis may have contributed to the improvement in symptoms.

*Acupuncture* One study of twenty-seven patients who received acupuncture treatments three times per week for two weeks found improvements in their quality of life and gastrointestinal-symptom scores. The results were the same as those observed among a comparison group that received relaxation training. However, the patients who received the acupuncture were more likely to see their pain reduction persist over the course of a four-week follow-up.

*Biofeedback* A mind/body technique in which participants see and realize their body's response to stimuli such as pain, biofeedback's proponents believe that it helps people modify their body's responses to these stimuli. With visual devices and easy instructions, patients can be taught how to alter such apparently automatic responses as the skin's temperature, for example, by altering the flow of blood to it. Some patients who have lost control of their bowels have been trained to better control them using biofeedback techniques to change the sphincter muscle's ability to contract. In one study, conducted at the University of Tennessee in Memphis, a biofeedback technique developed by NASA as a therapy for motion sickness was found to be effective for constipation. Study participants said that their symptoms—nausea, vomiting, abdominal pain, and gas—improved after just three sessions. Some say the technique works especially well for cramping.

*Herbal remedies* A number of herbs and other natural substances are being used by a growing portion of patients in pursuit of relief from IBS symptoms. Among the most popular substances are St. John's wort, fish oils, flaxseed oil, aloe vera juice, and a variety of Chinese herbs. Unfortunately, there are few studies to gauge the effectiveness of any of these remedies. A new product, however, made from fish protein, was found in one study to significantly reduce some IBS symptoms.

*Psychotherapy* Experts disagree on whether formal psychoanalysis is helpful in combating IBS. However, talking things out with an experienced and realistic therapist may help patients reduce stress and provide coping skills that improve mental health and associated physical ailments. In a 1983 Swedish study, IBS patients who combined medical treatment with individual psychotherapy showed more short-term and long-term improvement than those who had only medical therapy. A possible benefit of psychotherapy may be the discovery by the patient that he or she is depressed and that the depression is either a cause or result of IBS.

The important thing to remember throughout all searches for diagnoses and remedies is that every IBS patient is unique and that treatments should be tailored to the specific symptoms and needs of each individual. The good news is that IBS poses no threat to your life—with the right attitude and therapy techniques, patients can learn to live with irritable bowel syndrome while experiencing a minimum of interruption to their daily lives.

# 5

# Diseases with Symptoms Similar to Irritable Bowel Syndrome

Despite assurances that they have the relatively harmless irritable bowel syndrome (IBS), some people still worry that a more dangerous, perhaps life-threatening condition has somehow been missed. After all, there are a number of gastrointestinal diseases that can cause nonspecific symptoms that overlap with those of IBS. Fortunately, each has its own special characteristics that should serve as red flags to patients and doctors alike.

The four that will be addressed here include diverticular disease, Crohn's disease, ulcerative colitis, and colorectal cancer. Crohn's disease and ulcerative colitis are often referred to as inflammatory bowel disease and will be addressed as such here.

## Diverticular Disease

In patients affected by diverticular disease, small, fingerlike sacs or pouches protrude off the colon's inner lining, forming where the blood vessels that provide nutrition and oxygen to the colon enter the bowel. The sacs pierce the colon wall, causing areas of weakness.

Although the condition most commonly occurs after the age of fifty, anyone can develop these diverticula, and those who do are said to have diverticulosis. Fifty percent of people over age fifty have diverticulosis. In most cases, the colon does not become inflamed or infected, and there are no symptoms. Some persons with diverticulosis may experience bowel irregularity and abdominal cramping suggestive of IBS.

There are times, however, when the diverticula become inflamed or infected, due to perforations in the sacs that can appear as either large holes or microscopic ones (*see* Figure 5.1). This condition is called diverticulitis. Some symptoms can be similar to those in IBS: nausea and vomiting, constipation, or cramping.

Usually, however, the symptoms of diverticulitis are much more intense than IBS symptoms and include severe

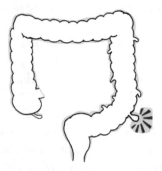

**FIGURE 5.1: DIVERTICULAR DISEASE**

lower-left abdominal pain, chills, fever, and an elevated white–blood cell count. In fact, these symptoms may mimic those of an inflamed appendix. When diverticula become severely inflamed, the colon can be obstructed or its wall can be perforated, resulting in peritonitis, a potentially dangerous inflammation of the membrane lining of the abdominal cavity.

No one knows how or why a diverticulum becomes inflamed, but it may be that dry, hard stool gets stuck in one of the sacs, allowing the bacteria there to proliferate in the damaged tissue and form an abscess.

The diagnosis of diverticulitis is made after a number of tests, among them usually a computerized tomographic (CT) scan. Treatment involves putting the patient on a liquid diet to let the bowel rest and beginning antibiotic therapy to clear the infection. After the acute infection has stabilized, patients are put on a steady high-fiber diet to help prevent flare-ups. Patients are also advised to avoid small nuts and seeds, which are hard to digest and tend to get caught in the crevices of the colon wall, thus possibly triggering an inflammation.

Recurring attacks of diverticulitis, the presence of a fistula (an abnormal tubelike passage that may occur between the sigmoid colon and the bladder, between the large intestine and small intestine, or from the intestine to the abdominal wall), or an abscess may require surgical resectioning of the colon.

## Inflammatory Bowel Disease

Inflammatory bowel disease (IBD) refers to chronic disorders in which the intestine becomes inflamed, often causing recurring abdominal cramps and diarrhea. The two main types are Crohn's disease and ulcerative colitis, which have many similarities and are therefore sometimes difficult to distinguish from each other. The causes of the diseases are not known. While the two diseases are often lumped together as inflammatory bowel disease and are treated in similar ways, physicians regard them as separate and distinct. Between 1 million and 2 million people in the United States have some form of IBD.

A chronic inflammatory condition of the gastrointestinal tract, inflammatory bowel disease affects a diverse population with a wide variety of symptoms that include chronic abdominal pain, diarrhea, rectal bleeding, fever, and weight loss. Some patients experience periods of fairly good health interrupted by flare-ups. Others experience continuous symptoms marked by serious inflammation, intestinal bleeding, and abdominal pain. The illness can also affect organs outside the gastrointestinal tract as well, as when inflammation extends from the bowel to block the ureter or cause hip inflammation, and can be tied to a host of problems, such as arthritis, liver disease, and eye and skin conditions. Both Crohn's disease and ulcerative colitis can cause pain in the joints, inflammation of the whites of the eyes, inflamed skin nodules, skin sores, and inflammation of the spine and pelvic joints. In addition, ulcerative colitis in particular is known to cause liver disease, including hepatitis, inflammation of the bile ducts, and cirrhosis. Many of these problems may result from the inflamed intestine's release of proteins called antigens, against which the body forms antibodies. The antigens and antibodies join together, travel in the circulation, and settle in various organs, thereby causing difficulties.

## Crohn's Disease

Crohn's disease is a chronic inflammation of the walls of the gastrointestinal (GI) tract. The cause isn't known, although researchers suspect that genetically determined dysfunction of the immune system, infection, or diet may be at its root. This inflammatory disease can occur anywhere in the GI tract, from the mouth to the anus, but is usually found in the lower part of the tract (*see* Figure 5.2). The inflammation involves the full thickness of the bowel wall, not just the inner lining, and may extend beyond the bowel to affect nearby organs. The bowel walls become thickened as well as chronically inflamed, and leakage of intestinal contents from the bowel via fistulae can cause internal abscesses and infections. Such fistulae are abnormal connections or passageways between parts of the intestine and other organs, and even, particularly near the anus, the skin surface. They allow intestinal contents to move from the intestine into areas, such as the bladder, where they can cause complications, including infections.

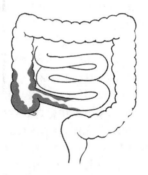

**FIGURE 5.2: CROHN'S DISEASE**

Crohn's disease usually appears in young people, and may first be noticed through pain in the right side of the abdomen, a low-grade fever, and perhaps changes in bowel movements. Some patients may lose weight (in children, growth may be delayed) and show a tender mass when the abdomen is palpated, distension from an obstructed bowel, blood in the stool, and non-gut manifestations such as arthritis, mouth sores, and painful red lumps on arms or legs—a rash called erythema nodosum. Some patients may develop an abscess or fistula around the rectum. Despite the possibility of abscesses and fistulae, however, severe bleeding is not a hallmark of Crohn's disease. Moreover, Crohn's disease accompanied by abdominal discomfort, tenderness, and diarrhea can resemble symptoms of irritable bowel syndrome and may often lead to diagnostic confusion.

## Ulcerative Colitis

This inflammatory bowel disease is characterized by damage to the lining, or mucosa, of the colon (*see* Figure 5.3), as opposed to Crohn's disease, in which the damage extends into the deeper layers of the intestinal wall. As in irritable bowel syndrome, there can be lower-abdominal pain and diarrhea; unlike with IBS, the stool generally contains blood, and bowel symptoms may be accompanied by fever, weight loss, an elevated white-blood-cell count, and the same non-gut manifestations as exhibited in Crohn's disease: arthritis, mouth sores, and erythema nodosum. Ulcerative colitis is easier to diagnose and to treat than Crohn's disease; it can even be cured because it affects only the colon, which can be surgically removed. Following removal of the colon, the end of the small intestine may empty through the skin of the abdominal wall as an "ileostomy," or, if possible, be fashioned into a "pouch" and hooked up to the anus as an ileal pouch—anal anastomosis.

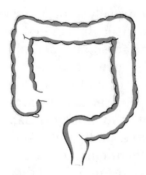

**FIGURE 5.3: ULCERATIVE COLITIS**

A number of tests are usually performed in diagnosing inflammatory bowel disease, but evidence of telltale inflammation of the colon can usually be seen via a colonoscopy or barium enema, allowing for a definitive diagnosis of the disease. An upper GI series with X rays of the small bowel can detect Crohn's disease of the small intestine.

Although the cause of IBD is not known, genetic factors are believed to play a role: 10 to 40 percent of people with IBD also have family members with the condition, and a gene that confers susceptibility to Crohn's disease has been identified in 20 percent of affected persons. Bacteria, environment, and diet may also be factors.

As for treatment of IBD, surgical removal of the colon is the only true cure for ulcerative colitis, but the illness varies in severity and surgery is too drastic a treatment for most patients with the disease. Crohn's disease cannot be cured with surgery, but in some cases surgery is needed to treat a complication of the disease, such as bowel obstruction. Meanwhile, although drugs cannot cure IBD, they are effective in reducing inflammation and accompanying symptoms in about 80 percent of patients. The drugs used most commonly are aminosalicylates (cousins of aspirin), steroids (potent anti-inflammatory agents), other immunosuppressants such as azathioprine (Imuran), and antibiotics.

A new drug, infliximab (Remicade), has proven effective for patients with Crohn's disease. Administered via infusion, the drug is an antibody that blocks a protein called tumor necrosis factor-alpha (TNF-alpha) that appears to cause the destruction of tissue.

In trials, up to 80 percent of patients taking Remicade showed evidence of improvement compared to only 16 percent given a placebo. Moreover, 48 percent of patients on the drug went into remission, compared to 4 percent of those on placebo. Remicade is considered an important advance and is the first of a number of similar drugs in development for treatment of Crohn's disease.

About 20 percent of patients with ulcerative colitis eventually have surgery to remove their colons. Roughly 70 percent of those with Crohn's disease eventually need surgery to remove damaged areas of their colons or small intestines. The most serious complication of IBD is colon cancer. The risk of colon cancer is much higher for patients with IBD than for the general population.

## Colorectal Cancer

Everyone's greatest fear is developing cancer, and colorectal cancer is the third most common form of cancer in both men and women *(see* Figure 5.4). An estimated 132,000 new cases are diagnosed each year in the United States.

For many people, any bowel irregularity is enough to start the mind worrying, however irrationally, about the worst-case scenario. Sometimes, the intestinal symptoms typifying irritable bowel syndrome may also be present with colon cancer; abdominal pain, cramping, bloating, gas pains, and changes in bowel patterns, for example, often accompany each condition. And blood in the stool or rectal bleeding—possible symptoms of inflammatory bowel disease—are also often present in colon cancer. Advanced can-

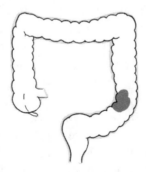

FIGURE 5.4: COLORECTAL CANCER

cer is likely to cause bloody bowel movements, severe constipation if the intestine is obstructed, and weight loss. That's why it is so important to be checked without delay if these symptoms manifest themselves.

The good news is that colon cancer can be prevented through screening. Almost all polyps can be spotted and removed during a colonoscopy. Even early-stage, localized colon cancer is curable in 90 percent of cases. To catch polyps or early cancer, the American Cancer Society recommends that, beginning at age fifty, men and women have one of the following at advised intervals: a fecal occult blood test (FOBT) and flexible sigmoidoscopy, colonoscopy, or double-contrast barium enema. A digital rectal exam should be done at the same time as each of these procedures. The FOBT should be repeated annually, the sigmoidoscopy every five years, and the colonoscopy every ten years. Likewise, the barium enema should be repeated every five to ten years. If an FOBT is positive or if a sigmoidoscopy or barium enema shows a polyp, a full colonoscopy should then be done.

# 6

# Constipation

*It is best when the stools are soft and passed at an hour customary to the patient when in health.*
—Hippocrates

Constipation means different things to different people. One thing is clear, however: it is a problem that seems to bother an awful lot of folks. In fact, constipation is one of the most common gastrointestinal complaints in the United States, responsible for more than 2.5 million visits to doctors each year. Experts say that it afflicts some 20 percent of the population on an ongoing basis, is more common in women than men, and usually increases with age.

But what, exactly, is constipation? Despite the magnitude of the problem, it is not an easy thing to define—although most people can probably tell you when they think they are constipated.

## How It Happens

Constipation is loosely defined as the slow movement of feces through the large intestine that results in the passage of dry, hard stool. It can cause discomfort and pain.

To understand constipation, it helps to know how the colon, or large intestine, works. As residue from the small intestine passes into and moves through the colon, the colon absorbs water while solidifying the waste products, or stool. Muscle contractions in the colon push the stool toward the rectum. By the time it gets to the rectum, the stool is solid because most of the water has been absorbed.

The hard, dry stool that characterizes constipation occurs when too much water is absorbed by the colon. This may happen because the muscle contractions of the colon are too slow or sluggish, causing the stool to move along too slowly. Conscious actions on the part of people who may try to delay a bowel movement can also play a role in causing constipation.

Bacteria constitute about a third of fecal solids and undigested material makes up another third. The rest consists of sloughed material from the intestine. As water is absorbed, the feces becomes increasingly compact as it moves down toward the rectum, propelled by muscle contractions (*see* Figure 6.1). When the fecal mass reaches the rectum, the last segment of the colon, it stays there until a sufficient volume accumulates and triggers the defecation reflex. It's possible to override the urge to defecate by consciously constricting the external sphincter, a group of muscles under voluntary control that surrounds the anus. If the process of active resistance becomes routine, there may be a blunting of the reflex to defecate. Accumulated stool may harden and become even more difficult to pass as a result.

Eventually, the colon tries to move the stool by squeezing down to the size of a pencil and then pushing it. This

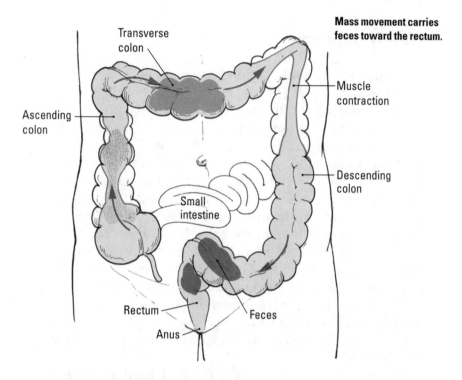

**Mass movement carries feces toward the rectum.**

Transverse colon

Ascending colon

Muscle contraction

Descending colon

Small intestine

Rectum

Feces

Anus

## FIGURE 6.1: HOW THE COLON WORKS

Fluid and indigestible particles flow from the small to the large intestine at their junction in the lower-right corner of the abdomen. Slow, churning motions move this material from the cecum along the ascending segment of the colon. In this phase, fluids and minerals are normally absorbed. Feces solidify in the transverse section of the colon and are propelled down the descending segment toward the rectum by periodic, firm muscle contractions.

causes an uncomfortable pressure and results in cramping. If the stool is not evacuated, more hard stool accumulates. When the stool finally passes the anus, it can cause extreme discomfort.

# Frequency of Bowel Movements: What's Normal?

It's no secret that some people are obsessed with their bowel movements. In fact, plenty of people are, as evidenced by the fact that Americans spend more than $400 million every year on laxatives in a bid to stay "regular."

But what is regularity? It's a concept probably based on a myth handed down throughout history: you've got to move your bowels each day to be healthy. Experts say that's bunk. In fact, as far back as 1909, the British physiologist Sir Arthur Hurst said that it was not unusual to find healthy people who had moved their bowels three times a day—or once every three days. Today, that's still the range of what's considered "normal."

Certainly, though, many perfectly healthy people don't fall within that range. In 1813, the British physician William Heberden described a patient who "never went but once a month." He also described a patient who relieved himself twelve times a day. Both patients seemed perfectly content with their bowel habits. The world's record for continence is held by a man who didn't move his bowels for 368 days in a case described by W. Grant Thompson in *Gut Reactions: Understanding Symptoms of the Digestive Tract.* That, of course, is far outside the range of normalcy. But the man survived, eventually delivering thirty-six liters of feces on the 369th day. Needless to say, there was much rejoicing when he finally did.

The truth is, we all experience variations in how often we go to the bathroom. Menstruation, vigorous physical exercise, diet, travel, stress—they all can cause temporary changes in bowel habits. Going a day without a bowel movement certainly should not be considered constipation. And three movements in a day is not necessarily diarrhea. In most cases, people should focus not on how often they go, but on the consistency of the stools they pass, the effort needed to expel them, any associated symptoms, and any severe changes in frequency before they think about seeking treatment.

According to one study, 20 to 40 percent of individuals said they strain while moving their bowels. But the study did not specify what "straining" meant. In laymen's terms, though, you may be constipated if you:

☞ Defecate less than three times a week and pass hard stool
☞ Strain from one to three out of four times you move your bowels
☞ Experience abdominal bloating or discomfort

The latest definition of functional constipation includes experiencing at least two of the following during any three-month period:

☞ Straining during more than one-quarter of bowel movements
☞ Passing lumpy or hard stools during more than one-quarter of bowel movements
☞ Having a sensation of incomplete evacuation in more than one-quarter of bowel movements
☞ Having a sensation that your rectum or anus is blocked during more than one-quarter of bowel movements.
☞ Resorting to manual maneuvers such as using a finger to help facilitate movement during more than one-quarter of bowel movements
☞ Fewer than three defecations per week

## Causes of Constipation

There are numerous causes of constipation, some of which can easily be prevented by improving one's habits and lifestyle and others that have to do with physiological problems and diseases.

Some of the more common causes of constipation include:

*Not enough fiber in the diet.* A diet too low in fiber (found in fruits, vegetables, and grains) and too high in fats (like those found in meats and cheeses) is the most common cause of constipation. The bulk and soft texture of fiber help prevent hard, dry stools that are difficult to pass. On average, Americans eat about five to twenty grams of fiber a day, well below the twenty to thirty-five grams recommended by the American Dietetic Association. One reason we get too little fiber is that we eat too many refined and processed foods from which the natural fiber has been removed in preparation.

Low-fiber diets also play a role in the very real problem of constipation among the elderly. Older people sometimes lack interest in eating and, because they are convenient and cheap, choose fast foods that also happen to be low in fiber. Lack of teeth may also prompt elderly people to eat soft processed foods that are low in fiber.

In other parts of the world, particularly Africa, where people live primarily on diets with high vegetable and grain content, constipation is rare.

*Not enough liquids.* Water, juice, and other liquids are critical too, adding fluid to the colon and bulk to the stool, making bowel movements softer and easier to move along. Most people should drink about eight eight-ounce glasses of these liquids per day. Still, there is no reason to overdo it. Most people's fluid requirements are tied directly to their thirst level, so if their thirst is satisfied, they're probably getting enough fluids. Drinking more won't help constipation go away because fluids can't wash out the colon—the small intestine absorbs most of the liquid. So, trying to liquify hard stools by drinking more water or other fluids usually won't work unless your intake of liquids has been much too low to start with. Also, certain liquids, such as those containing caffeine, may have a dehydrating effect that can be counterproductive, although some people say that drinking coffee seems to help them move their bowels.

## Lack of Exercise

People who exercise regularly rarely complain about constipation. Sometimes, running or jogging, for example, will actually trigger a bowel movement—although, fortunately, not right there on the spot.

Basically, the colon responds to activity. It isn't going to move if you don't. This is quite clear when you examine people who are confined to bed rest after, say, an accident or surgery: bed rest is simply disastrous on the bowels. It's one reason why efforts are often made to get the elderly out of their beds and into an exercise program, even a modest one.

Good muscle tone in general is important to regular bowel movements. The abdominal wall muscles and the diaphragm both play a critical role in the process of defecation. If these muscles are flabby, they're not going to be able to do the job as well.

## Medications

Taking any one of a number of prescription or over-the-counter drugs can bring constipation as a side effect. Pain medications, especially narcotics, antacids that contain aluminum, antispasmodics, antidepressants, tranquilizers and sedatives, bismuth salts, iron supplements, diuretics, anticholinergics, calcium-channel blockers, and anticonvulsants for epilepsy are among those that can cause constipation.

People who begin experiencing persistent constipation for no apparent reason should consider the possibility that the cause may be any medications they may have recently begun taking. Drugs that are taken to control high blood pressure, for example, can affect colon motility. Iron can cause the stool to become dark and induce cramps along with constipation. Anticholinergics, sometimes used to manage irritable bowel syndrome (IBS), can inhibit the motor activity of the stomach, small bowel, and colon. Many commonly used antidepressants have anticholinergic properties, so they, too, can cause constipation. Some drugs used to treat Parkinson's disease can cause constipation as well.

Certain opiates, such as morphine, were actually used to treat diarrhea before they were given to control pain. Morphine delays gastric emptying and kills the urge to have a bowel movement.

## Irritable Bowel Syndrome

Some people who suffer from irritable bowel syndrome—sometimes called spastic colon—have spasms in the colon that affect bowel movements. In patients with irritable bowel syndrome, constipation and diarrhea often alternate, and cramping, gas, and bloating are common symptoms. (For more on irritable bowel syndrome, *see* Chapter 4, Irritable Bowel Syndrome.)

## Abuse of Laxatives

Myths about constipation, in some cases, have led to serious laxative abuse, particularly in the elderly, many of whom believe that their bowels must be moved at least once a day. In addition, some people with eating disorders, particularly young women, use laxatives to lose weight. This is a very dangerous practice. A British survey of London factory workers and patients of rural physicians (comprising a total of some 1,455 persons, deemed representative of the overall British population) showed that 20 percent used laxatives, even though many of them claimed not to be constipated.

People who use laxatives for a long time often come to rely on them for both psychological and physiological reasons; the colon may begin to rely on laxatives to spur bowel movements. In time, it is possible that laxatives can damage nerve cells in the colon and inhibit the colon's innate ability to contract. Stimulant laxatives, in particular, have been thought to decrease the force of intestinal contractions over time. These laxatives irritate the bowel to make it contract vigorously and expel water. On the good side, currently used laxatives appear to be safer than those used in the past. (For more, *see* box, Oral Laxatives, pp. 116–17).

## Changes in Life or Routine

Change your regular routine and you risk changing your bowel habits.

Pregnancy, for example, may cause women to become constipated because of hormonal changes or because the heavy uterus pushes on the intestine. Aging often affects regularity because a slower metabolism can cause less intestinal activity and reduce muscle tone.

Traveling can also cause some people to become backed up because it means an alteration in normal diet and daily routines. While most travelers fear diarrhea when they visit a foreign land, traveler's constipation can be nearly as much of a nuisance for some. Traveler's constipation can occur even in clean, modern countries, such as those of Europe, in contrast to traveler's diarrhea, which is most common in Third World countries.

Europeans, in fact, often complain about traveler's constipation when visiting the United States. This might result from the American diet or a disorientation similar to jet lag: a person has changed time zones, but the body hasn't caught up. Usually, the condition goes away in a few days, but it's not unusual for it to last a week or two. Once the bowels resume working, they usually continue to do so, although some travelers pack a laxative in their kits just in case.

## Ignoring the Urge

If you have to go, go. If you hold in a bowel movement, for whatever reason, you may be inviting a bout of constipation. People who repeatedly ignore the urge to move their bowels may eventually stop feeling the urge.

Why would someone ignore the urge? There are lots of reasons. Perhaps they are not near a toilet or don't want to use a public toilet out of shyness, fear of germs, or other concerns. Let's face it: some public toilets—those in many service stations along the highway, for example—are perfectly disgusting. Many reasonable people may want to take a pass and wait for a more inviting facility.

Some people may simply postpone evacuation because they are too busy or are under emotional strain. Some children simply don't like to go to the bathroom because of lingering psychological problems stemming from a stressful toilet training or because they don't want to interrupt a game of ball.

For whatever reason, however, it's not a good idea to ignore the urge.

## Some Diseases Can Cause Constipation

A number of diseases are known to cause constipation, so a newly developed constipation problem may result from the progression of an underlying illness.

Diseases that can cause constipation include neurological disorders, such as Parkinson's disease, spinal cord injury, stroke, and multiple sclerosis; metabolic and endocrine disorders, such as hypothyroidism, diabetes, and chronic kidney failure; and bowel cancer and diverticulitis (see Chapter 5, Diseases with Symptoms Similar to Irritable Bowel Syndrome). A number of systemic conditions that affect organ systems, lupus and scleroderma among them, can also cause constipation.

Any of these disorders can slow the movement of stool through the colon, rectum, or anus. In addition, intestinal obstructions, caused by scar tissue (adhesions) from a prior operation or strictures of the colon or rectum, can compress, squeeze, or narrow the intestine and rectum, causing constipation.

## Chronic, Severe Constipation

In rare cases, some people experience persistent constipation for years or decades, even though they have no physical abnormality of the bowel. The condition is known as functional constipation or chronic ideopathic constipation. Those with chronic severe constipation do not respond to standard treatments and may not improve despite reasonable efforts to change their diet and adjust toilet habits.

Most common in women, chronic constipation may be related to problems with hormone control or with the muscles and nerves in the colon, rectum, or anus. These people may have what is known as colonic inertia (sluggish colon) or, less commonly, anorectal dysfunction—for example, the paradoxical contraction of the pelvic muscles and internal anal sphincter when they should relax. Colonic inertia may affect the entire colon or may be limited to the left or lower (sigmoid) colon. Anorectal dysfunction results from an inability to relax the rectal and anal muscles to allow stool to leave.

# Hirschsprung's Disease

A rare type of constipation, Hirschsprung's disease stems from a problem in the neural connections in the wall of the lower bowel, most often in the rectum. The result is that one part of the rectum remains narrowed and contracted and fails to open properly. The disease usually occurs early in infancy and causes severe constipation. If not diagnosed, it may lead to a condition in which the colon dilates to a huge size, becoming a megacolon. Most people with the condition have had problems moving their bowels from infancy. The condition can be repaired surgically.

# Screening and Diagnosis

Diagnosing constipation may sound simple, but if a doctor wants to find out what's causing the problem, particularly if it persists, that will involve taking a medical history and performing a physical exam.

The physical exam may involve a visual examination and feeling of the abdomen for any unusual masses or tenderness, as well as a digital rectal exam to feel for polyps or other abnormalities and to assess the strength of the anal sphincter muscle. Reviewing any medications that may be contributing to the problem is also important. If such medications are not found to be the cause of the problem, any one of several further tests may help determine if there is a blockage in the colon or an underlying condition such as hypothyroidism.

Among the tests that might be ordered are a fecal occult blood test to determine whether there is blood in the stool; a barium enema, or a sigmoidoscopy or colonoscopy, to look for polyps or other irregularities. For patients with severe long-standing constipation, special tests, including a colonic transit study (to measure the speed of passage of food from the beginning to the end of the colon), defecography (an X ray of the rectum, taken as barium paste is evacuated), and anorectal manometry (measurement of the pressure of anal contraction), may be required.

## The Wonders of Fiber

The most important thing you can do to prevent constipation or to treat it if it occurs is to add plenty of fiber to your diet. It has been well known since ancient times that bran serves to expand and soften the stool. Indeed, in 430 B.C., Hippocrates himself noted that while "white bread is more nutritious; it makes less feces" than "wholemeal bread [which] cleans out the gut and passes through as excrement." Bran will also hurry gastrointestinal transit in people whose movement is slow, but at least twenty grams of unprocessed bran per day is necessary to do so. Depending on the brand, a bowl of bran cereal will provide anywhere from four to twelve grams of fiber. Bran is one of two types of dietary fiber that may be helpful in treating constipation. Known as insoluble fiber, bran appears to act as a laxative by adding bulk to the stool.

Bran may be consumed in muffins, bread, or cereals, or sprinkled over food or stirred into juice. Doctors recommend starting with one teaspoon per meal, increasing slowly until the proper result is obtained. Fiber works in part by absorbing water and swelling, so be sure to drink water or other liquids along with it. Be warned, however: in some people, bran can instead "plug" the bowel. For such people who cannot tolerate large amounts of bran, insoluble fiber can also be found in methylcellulose supplements such as Citrucel, which makes stool softer.

The other type of fiber that may help treat constipation is soluble fiber. Psyllium or the pectins in fruit are considered soluble fiber, meaning that they retain water and, as a result, bulk up and soften the stool. Some soluble fiber is also digested by colon bacteria, which then create gas and help to increase fecal mass. Fiber in general also speeds up transit time and lowers pressure in the lower colon, possibly allowing the contents to pass through faster and more easily. The packaged psyllium sold in drugstores is, for all intents and purposes, a dietary supplement and is considered safe for long-term use. Among the most popular psyllium products are Metamucil and Fiberall.

Of course, it may not be necessary for a constipated person to load up on bran or fiber supplements. Simply eating plenty of raw fruits and vegetables may do the job for many people (see box, Good Sources of Dietary Fiber). Besides fiber content, some foods, such as prunes and figs, contain natural substances that spur intestinal evacuation.

## GOOD SOURCES OF DIETARY FIBER

| INSOLUBLE FIBER | SOLUBLE FIBER |
| --- | --- |
| Wheat bran | Oat bran |
| Corn bran | Whole oats |
| Whole grains | Rice bran |
| Dried beans and peas | Dried beans |
| Popcorn | Chickpeas, black-eyed peas |
| Seeds and nuts | Lentils |
| Most fruits and vegetables, especially carrots, white potatoes, artichokes, broccoli leeks, parsnips | All fruits and vegetables, especially citrus fruits, apples, pears, sweet potatoes, carrots, okra, corn |

# Treatment

Beyond fiber, people suffering from constipation may try a number of measures, including boosting fluid intake and increasing physical exercise, in pursuit of relief. Drinking more fluids may reduce the need for the colon to rehydrate stools and is, in any case, harmless. And exercise, which is widely believed to promote regularity (although few studies have investigated this), has many other health benefits as well. Under most circumstances, laxatives should be used only when dietary and behavioral measures fail. That said, following is a discussion of various constipation treatments.

### Laxatives

Stimulant laxatives contain chemicals that act directly on the intestine to increase the secretion of water into the interior. Some of them also elicit more vigorous contractions from the colon. Using them daily over a period of months, however, can increase colonic peristalsis, possibly making the colon flabby, inert, and always in need of a chemical "fix." Called "lazy bowel syndrome," this condition is less common now than in the past (*see* box, Oral Laxatives). For those who have lost the sensations that remind them to move their bowels, though, only the use of laxatives may do the job.

---

## ORAL LAXATIVES

All laxatives increase the bulk and water content of stool as well as soften it, although they probably achieve these effects in different ways.

☛ **Bulk-forming agents** are thought to be safe to take indefinitely on a daily basis. They include:

- Bran (in food and supplements)
- Calcium polycarbophil
- Methylcellulose (in products such as Citrucel, Cologel)
- Psyllium (in products such as Metamucil and others)

- **Stool softeners** merge with feces and soften their consistency, but they can have other effects.

  - Docusate (Colace, Dialose, Surfak, others) is generally safe for long-term use.

  - Mineral oil reduces absorption of fat-soluble vitamins and can produce lung damage if accidentally inhaled. Daily use is discouraged.

- **Osmotic agents** are salts or carbohydrates that promote secretion of water into the colon. They are reasonably safe, even with prolonged use.

- **Chemical stimulants** can lead to dependency, have diminished effects with daily use over months or years, and may cause changes in the bowel over time. However, they are often effective when used once or twice for occasional constipation.

  - Bisacodyl (in Dulcolax, Correctol, Feen-A-Mint, for example)
  - Casanthranol (included in Dialose Plus, Peri-Colace)
  - Cascara (included in Nature's Remedy)
  - Castor oil (in Neoloid, Purge)
  - Senna (in Ex-Lax, Fletcher's Castoria, Senokot, and other products)

---

Most laxatives are available in liquid, tablet, gum, and powder forms. A plant laxative, senna, has been used for generations in the form of a tea. It is available in many products, one of them being Senokot.

In some cases, your doctor may recommend a stool softener or lubricant, such as mineral oil or docusate sodium (Colace), to soften fecal matter so it moves through the intestines more easily. However, these can occasionally cause problems if used on a long-term basis. Lubricants such as mineral oil are generally frowned upon because they can be habit forming and may interfere with the absorption of vitamins. Moreover, if mineral oil is inhaled into the lungs, it can cause pneumonia. The prolonged use of docusate sodium may, in rare cases, result in liver damage.

Laxatives pose special concerns during pregnancy. Pregnant women should avoid any laxatives other than fiber supplements without a physician's okay. Furthermore, those taking iron supplements, or prenatal supplements high in iron, should ask their doctor about reducing the dose, since iron can be very constipating for some people.

### Suppositories

Suppositories have been used to aid evacuation since the days of ancient Egypt, Greece, and Rome. Glycerine suppositories are made up of about 70 percent glycerine, sometimes with sodium stearate (a fatty acid) added. When inserted, a glycerine suppository draws water into the bowel from surrounding bowel tissues, providing a soft stool mass and increased bowel action. Suppositories with the stimulant bisacodyl (such as Dulcolax) are more potent stimulants of defecation and usually produce a bowel movement within fifteen to twenty minutes. They work by increasing the muscle contractions in the intestinal wall that move along the stool mass.

### Enemas

Like suppositories, enemas have been around since ancient times, and, like suppositories, they are usually used primarily when oral laxatives don't work. Pumping water into the colon works to stimulate defecation. The simple tap water enema distends the rectum, mimicking its natural distension by stool and thus prompts the reflex by which the rectum empties itself via the sphincters opening themselves.

While it isn't ideal to become dependent on artificial stimulation to kick off evacuation, an enema is probably the most benign way of doing so.

Although the tap water enema works just fine, compounds made up of sodium phosphates are available in single-dose plastic containers. These salts attract an outpouring of fluid into the bowel, prompting bowel contraction. Oil-containing enemas are sometimes prescribed as softeners for feces that have become hardened within the rectum. They are generally recommended for short-term use only.

### Other Dietary Approaches

Some people recommend eating pine nuts, flaxseed, or sesame seeds to ease a mild case of constipation, claiming these foods' lubricating effect can help. The idea is to eat a handful once a day, chewing thoroughly and washing it down with a glass of water. Also touted by many is apple juice, particularly when it is mixed with aloe vera juice. Proponents say it is best to drink the mix—four ounces of apple juice, four ounces of aloe vera—in the morning on an empty stomach—but drink just one glass per day.

### Massage

Boosters of massage say the rubbing technique can be helpful in easing constipation. The idea, basically, is to rub it out. Massage the abdomen in a circular motion about 100 times until the urge to go is felt. Another method is direct stimulation of the colon, which begins on the right side just over the hip bone and runs across the bottom of the rib cage to the left side, and down to the hip bone on that side. Massaging along that path, following the flow inside the colon, is said to help stimulate bowel movement.

## Acupressure

In the ancient disciplines of acupuncture and acupressure, there is said to be located in the web between the index finger and the thumb a pressure point for relieving constipation. Squeezing this point with the index finger and thumb of the other hand while breathing deeply is supposed to stimulate the urge to go.

## Bowel Retraining

For those who have gotten into the bad habit of suppressing the urge to defecate, a bowel retraining program may prove helpful. For such people, it may help to sit on a toilet, book or magazine in hand, for about twenty minutes each morning, right after breakfast, to encourage the return of reflexes that have disappeared. Straining, however, is a no-no, since it may lead to a tightening of muscles that should be relaxed for comfortable evacuation.

People with chronic constipation caused by anorectal dysfunction may want to try biofeedback to retrain the muscles that control the release of bowel movements. Biofeedback involves using a sensor that monitors muscle actions and simultaneously displays information about those actions on a monitor. The information may be used by the patient and doctor to help the patient learn how to use these muscles properly and gain control over muscles, such as the internal anal sphincter, that we don't generally have voluntary control over.

When trying to reestablish normal bowel function, it is important to have regular bowel habits. Try to have a bowel movement at the same time each day. The colon is usually most active after a person wakes up or eats, so right after breakfast may be the best time to try. Comfortable surroundings may help as well; nobody is going to be successful trying to move his or her bowels in a cold, drafty room, for example. Also, squatting is considered the best position for evacuation. Use a footstool in front of the toilet to elevate the feet or bend forward so that your abdomen rests against your thighs. If you feel stool in the rectum but can't get it out, try pushing from the outside, using your hand placed in front of the rectum or just behind it.

There may be a psychological component to bowel retraining, too. For example, some people insist that they can't move their bowels unless they have their morning cigarette or cup of coffee. And some people can use only the toilet in their own home or can go only if they are alone in the house. Such phobias may need to be addressed in therapy.

## Medications

Studies of two experimental drugs, prucalopride and tegaserod, have shown them to be effective in treating chronic constipation due to slow motility. Known as $5\text{-HT}_4$ receptor antagonists, these drugs are designed to stimulate the $5\text{-HT}_4$ receptors on cholinergic nerves—key moderators of the nervous system—in the muscles of the colon. Prucalopride and tegaserod bind to the $5\text{-HT}_4$ receptors, provoking the release of neurotransmitters and inducing peristalsis, the intestinal contractions that move matter through the bowel. In one study, prucalopride was found to increase the frequency of bowel movements from fewer than two per week to more than three per week in about one-third of patients. However, a distantly related drug, alosetron (Lotronex), which worked against the $5\text{-HT}_3$ receptor and had been approved for treatment of diarrhea in irritable bowel syndrome patients, was pulled from the market after patients using it experienced severe, even life-threatening, complications including ischemic colitis and acute constipation. One patient needed to have her colon removed.

## Surgery

Thanks to dismal results, surgical intervention to treat severe constipation, even after all else has failed, has fallen far out of fashion. The operation involves surgically removing the colon, with the idea being to sacrifice the large bowel and connect the small intestine directly to the rectum. At least half of all those undergoing the procedure, however, have had to endure further surgery because of small-bowel obstructions. Some say the surgery may be suitable for people with colonic inertia, but not for those with constipation due to anorectal dysfunction. In any case, most surgeons resort to surgery very rarely.

## Complications

Although most cases of constipation can be treated by using one or more of the methods described in this chapter, stubborn constipation can sometimes lead to physiological complications.

Hemorrhoids, for example, can be caused by straining to produce a bowel movement. They consist of a mass of dilated vascular "cushions" in swollen tissue at the anus or just within the rectum. They can bleed or cause severe discomfort. And anal fissures (tears in the skin around the anus) can occur when hard stool stretches the sphincter muscle beyond its capabilities. As a result, rectal bleeding may take place.

Treatment of hemorrhoids may include sitz baths (warm baths, sometimes with Epsom salts), ice packs, and applications of ointment to the affected area. Using stool softeners and fiber supplements is helpful too. Occasionally, surgery may be indicated. Anal fissures are treated by topical medications such as nitroglycerine or the injection of botulinum toxin, which relaxes the sphincter muscle. In some cases, stretching the sphincter muscle or surgically removing tissue or skin in the affected area is necessary.

Once in a while, straining can cause a tiny bit of the lining of the intestine to push out from the anus, a condition known as rectal prolapse. Usually, it can be made to reverse itself simply by stopping the straining. If not, surgery to strengthen and tighten the anal sphincter muscle or to repair the prolapsed lining may be necessary.

Severe constipation may also cause hard stool to pack the intestine and rectum so tightly that pushing cannot expel it, no matter what treatment is tried. This condition, called fecal impaction, usually requires the stool to be softened by an enema. Even then, a doctor may have to stick a finger or two into the anus and dig out the impacted stool, a perfectly disagreeable job if ever there was one. The condition, however, is serious, and may even become life-threatening if not resolved. Patients with fecal impaction may develop circulatory, cardiac, or respiratory disorders, for example.

# 7

# Diarrhea

*Eat what you want and let the food fight it out inside.*
—Mark Twain

The flip side of constipation, diarrhea is a condition in which bowel movements occur too frequently and stools are very loose and watery.

Although diarrhea can accompany a number of gastrointestinal disorders both functional and organic, it may also occur on its own, intermittently or chronically, for a number of reasons. But whether this miserable condition is the result of a virus, bacteria, the blue-plate special at the local greasy spoon, or the infamous Montezuma's revenge, it all means the same thing: it's the body saying no to whatever it is that has been introduced into the intestines.

Some believe that having more than three bowel movements a day constitutes diarrhea, but that definition is too inclusive for most experts. The more widely accepted definition of diarrhea is frequent liquid or watery stools. It is sometimes accompanied by cramping and abdominal pain before the dam bursts. When diarrhea occurs more than three-quarters of the time over a period of at least three months without an identifiable cause, it is said to be functional.

Regardless of how it's defined, when you've got diarrhea, you usually know it.

Although everybody experiences diarrhea sometimes, the condition is persistent for a significant percentage of the population. A British population survey, for example, showed that 5 percent of men and 4 percent of women experience liquid stools most of the time.

Diarrhea is the body's way of clearing from the intestines whatever is causing the upset. Sometimes, we can pinpoint exactly what it was that caused the intestinal distress. Other times, it remains a mystery, attributed perhaps to something "going around." In most cases, the problem will clear up on its own in a few days. We may not even have to call a doctor; home treatment may be all that is needed. Still, diarrheal illness is considered the second–most common clinical sickness in our society. Everyone gets it, from infants to the elderly, and when we do, it's something we want to get over as quickly as possible. Having "the runs," "the trots," or "Montezuma's revenge"—or whatever else we wish to call it—is no fun. Most times, we're able to control when we go. Other times . . . well, let's just say it helps to stay close to a toilet.

While diarrhea isn't usually serious, it certainly can be. Dehydration and weight loss are two common complications. Cases that don't clear up in a few days, or chronic or functional cases, will certainly require a doctor's care.

## Mechanisms of Diarrhea

Normal defecation depends on the small intestine, colon, rectum, and anal sphincter working in concert and as they are supposed to. When diarrhea strikes, it means that something has gone wrong.

The small intestine usually handles about eight liters of fluid per day from food and secretions, absorbing about seven and pushing about one liter to the colon. The colon absorbs most of that as it moves the compacted residue, which contains but a few ounces of water, to the rectum. The rectum can store up to 200 grams of normal stool before defecation is triggered.

Any interference with this process can cause the colon to be overwhelmed by the fluid load, resulting in diarrhea. In fact, any disturbance in the colon that interferes with the packing, storage, and drying-out of the stool can result in diarrhea. Some studies of functional diarrhea reveal that it might be caused in part by the feces moving too rapidly through the colon, too much fluid residue remaining in the small intestine, decreased colon contractions, or lessened anal-sphincter pressure. Another possible explanation for functional diarrhea is malfunction of the enteric nervous system, which controls the motor and secretory activities of the gut.

## Causes of Diarrhea

Everyday diarrhea can be caused by any one of a number of bacteria, viruses, or parasites entering the intestines, as well as by a number of foods, drugs, medical conditions, and treatments.

*Viruses* Any one of a number of viruses can cause diarrhea. Among them are the rhinovirus or adenovirus, rotavirus (the most common cause in infants), influenza, Norwalk agent (most common cause in adults), and a number of intestinal viruses. Cytomegalovirus and HIV are also known to cause diarrhea. Most of these viruses are spread by contaminated food or water, or by contaminated persons. Like with the common cold, little can be done to prevent infection aside from staying clear of those known to be sick with such viruses.

*Bacteria* A number of bacteria are associated with diarrhea. Among the most common are *Shigella, Salmonella,* cholera, *E. coli,* and *Campylobacter.* To prevent contracting diarrhea via a bacterial infection, the best method is to make sure that food is prepared safely. *E. coli* infection, for example, can be prevented by cooking meat thoroughly. Be sure as well to wash hands before handling raw meat or poultry, and clean all cutting boards, utensils, and countertops after they have come in contact with raw meat or poultry. And foods such as chicken, tuna, and macaroni salad should be refrigerated until just before they are eaten.

*Food poisoning* Usually, food poisoning is the culprit when more than one person experiences the same illness soon after eating the same food. Such cases are usually the result of any of the bacteria just noted getting into the food supply consumed by those who have fallen ill.

*Parasites* Intestinal parasites such as *Giardia lamblia, Cryptosporidium parvum,* and roundworms or tapeworms may also result in symptoms of diarrhea. Parasites are most often picked up by drinking contaminated water, although infected food handlers also pose a risk. Making sure that your drinking water is safe is one way to try to prevent the problem. There have been cases in which entire municipal water supplies have been contaminated; home water filters may help in such circumstances. Buying bottled water, however, is not necessarily a safe solution: just because the water is bottled is no guarantee that it will be free of infectious agents.

*Diseases of the bowel* Crohn's disease and ulcerative colitis, two forms of inflammatory bowel disease (IBD) *(see* Chapter 5, Diseases with Symptoms Similar to Irritable Bowel Syndrome) are associated with a number of symptoms, including diarrhea.

*Immune deficiency* Patients suffering from diseases such as AIDS or treatments for diseases such as cancer, which cause the immune system to be weakened, may also suffer from severe diarrhea.

*Stress* Emotions have been known to wreak havoc with the bowels in a number of ways. Diarrhea is a common complaint of those under severe stress or emotional upset.

*Foods* Certain foods, even if perfectly fresh, may result in diarrhea in some people. Among the usual—but by no means only—suspects are certain fruits, beans, and coffee. Of course, unripe fruits or spoiled foods of all types will likely cause diarrhea in most people, as will certain foods that a person cannot tolerate, such as milk products for those who are lactose intolerant.

*Medications* A number of drugs, prescription and over-the-counter alike, can cause diarrhea as a side effect. Among the worst culprits are antibiotics, antacids containing magnesium, and some blood pressure and heart medications. Antibiotics may also cause diarrhea by predisposing patients to a special type of bacterial infection, *Clostridium difficile*.

## Diagnosis

If your diarrhea is troublesome enough to warrant a trip to the doctor's office, he or she will likely take a medical history and perform a physical exam that probably will include a detailed examination of the abdomen. The doctor will want to make sure that you are in fact suffering from diarrhea and then decide if it is being caused by an organic problem, whether it is functional or chronic, or if it is simply the result of a virus or bacteria and is likely of short-term duration.

The history should include questions about the patient's habits, including drug or alcohol use. Alcohol abuse commonly results in diarrhea, for example, and the use of certain drugs, including cocaine, may also bring on diarrhea. The doctor will probably ask questions such as the following:

- When did the diarrhea start?
- Have any other family members been sick?
- Have you recently traveled out of the country?
- Are you experiencing abdominal pain? Fever? Chills?
- Is there blood in your stool?
- Is your diarrhea worse when you are under stress?
- Do any specific foods make it worse?
- Do you drink coffee? Alcohol?
- What medications are you taking or have you taken recently?

If diarrhea is accompanied by pus or blood in the stool, or if there is fever, anemia, loss of appetite, or vomiting, it is not likely a case of functional diarrhea.

For most people, and for most mild episodes of diarrhea, no specific lab tests are required. But for more severe forms, the doctor may order stool tests to look for pus cells that could indicate the presence of certain bacteria and to culture the causative bacteria. Blood may be drawn as well, to test for hemoglobin, white-cell count, and sedimentation rate. A sigmoidoscopy (examination of the rectum, sigmoid colon, and possibly descending colon with a flexible tube containing a tiny camera) may also be performed to look for organic diseases. For those over forty, a colonoscopy or a barium enema may be ordered in certain cases to check for organic diseases.

In seeking a diagnosis and deciding on a treatment for diarrhea, doctors must exclude the possibility of Crohn's disease or ulcerative colitis or other serious illness, even colon cancer. Often these are accompanied by blood in the stool, fever, and weight loss. In most cases, however, colon tumors do not cause chronic diarrhea.

## Prevention

Prevention of diarrhea is largely a matter of luck—and common sense. Diarrhea is often the result of a viral infection, and those are hard to avoid. However, using common sense—like knowing to stay away from children who are sick with diarrhea—is a good idea. If they are your children, though, that's obviously not possible.

Food is a great place to start diarrhea prevention. If certain foods give your intestinal tract a hard time, stay away from them. Make sure to wash fruits and vegetables well, and make sure they are ripe when you eat them. Clean chicken before you cook it, and be certain to cook chicken and other meats thoroughly. Clean all food preparation areas, such as countertops and cutting boards, well, and wash your hands thoroughly before and after handling food. (Do note, though, that the use of antibacterial soaps, cleaners, and sponges is controversial, as some infectious disease specialists say that their overuse can make the problem of antibiotic resistance worse for society.)

Be careful about eating foods left outside for long periods of time at barbecues or picnics: bacteria can grow easily in the warm air. And don't take leftovers home from these events. Even inside, leftovers should be refrigerated quickly after the meal has been served.

When dining out in restaurants, look around for clues as to cleanliness. It doesn't matter if you are in a four-star gourmet restaurant or a diner: If the bathroom is a mess, you probably don't want to eat there. Food servers, too, should look clean and neat. At a sushi bar, the glass partition that separates diners from the fish should be cold to the touch. Watch out for Caesar salads—they may be made with raw eggs, which can carry *Salmonella* or other bacteria. And chicken salad may be made from leftovers, a potential source of bacteria. If you take a doggie bag home from a restaurant, make sure you go straight home and not to a movie first, unless you have an ice chest in your car or the temperature outside is very cold.

## Traveler's Diarrhea

Some of the worst cases of diarrhea are those experienced every day by people who travel, particularly to Third World or developing countries. Usually, such attacks begin within a few days of arriving abroad or soon after returning home. You're one of the lucky ones if your traveler's diarrhea (TD) waits until you get home—at least you can be sick in familiar surroundings.

Such episodes can absolutely ruin a vacation or business trip. When TD occurs, you may experience cramps, bloating, nausea, a general sick feeling, and even fever. Sometimes, the diarrhea may be violent and frequent—an average five episodes of loose, watery stools a day. It may last three or four days to a week.

Although TD can occur in any country, it most often happens in those considered to be developing or Third World nations. This is because bacteria and the toxins that cause diarrhea occur in areas with contaminated water supplies, poor sewage systems, or inadequate food handling or preparation techniques, all of which are more prevalent in less-developed areas. In fact, studies show that 50 percent of tourists to developing countries experience diarrhea. High-risk destinations include Latin America, Africa, and the

Middle East. Mexico, of course, is notorious. The problem is most often experienced by younger tourists, perhaps because they are usually more adventurous in their eating than are older people.

For travelers, raw foods of all types are the most risky. Where one eats is also important, with food from street vendors being the most dangerous. And water, of course, is critical. Tap water should be avoided at all costs. Even using it to brush your teeth is risky: a single drop of contaminated water on a piece of lettuce, for example, can carry millions of TD-causing bacteria.

The problem is that travelers who enter a developing nation from a developed one experience a rapid change in the organisms that ordinarily inhabit the intestinal tract. Those who come down with TD ingest too much of the new infectious agents for their normal defense system to deal with. People living in those countries are already used to the bacteria, so they don't bother them at all. The most common of these bacteria is *E. coli*, which releases a toxin that causes the bowel to expel fluids and electrolytes, leading to dehydration. Other bacteria that are common culprits of TD are *Salmonella*, *Shigella*, and *Campylobacter*.

Fortunately, there are steps to help prevent traveler's diarrhea. First, adhere to the old adage, "If you can't cook it, boil it, or peel it, forget it." When avoiding the local tap water, don't forget about ice cubes. Putting ice cubes made from local tap water into your margarita is a sure recipe for disaster—it's better to drink the local bottled beer. And use bottled water for everything. If bottled water is not available, travelers can carry a portable water filter, or treat tap water by boiling it for ten minutes, or add one iodine tablet to a quart of water thirty minutes before drinking it.

While there are no vaccines to be had before leaving on your trip, travelers can help protect themselves by taking two tablets of Pepto Bismol four times a day before and during international travel. This can cut the risk of diarrhea by

60 percent, according to some studies. Such medication may also be started at the first sign of diarrhea. Some people take diphenoxylate (Lomotil) or loperamide (Imodium), which also appear to be effective. In addition, a few antibiotics, such as doxycycline (Vibramycin), trimethoprim/sulfamethoxazole (Bactrim, Septra) and ciprofloxacin (Cipro), have proven effective in reducing the risk of getting TD, but they carry side effects and are generally not advised. These side effects include rashes, allergic reactions, yeast infections in women, and an inclination to sunburn easily—not something you want if you're on a sun-and-fun vacation in Mexico or the Caribbean. An oral vaccine that kills *E. coli* is in development, as are vaccines for other common diarrhea-causing bacteria.

Research also suggests that an enzyme found in the stems of pineapples may also protect travelers against offending bacteria.

## Treatment

Most people with acute diarrhea can get over it on their own. It is generally self-limiting and runs its course in a few days. Even so, in many cases, particularly with severe or prolonged episodes of diarrhea, replacement of lost fluids and electrolytes (blood chemicals such as sodium and potassium) is essential to combat dehydration. Clear liquids are the first choice of means to do so. If you can't see through it, stay away from it. For mild cases of dehydration, clear or light-colored juices, regular (not diet) soft drinks, clear broth, and safe water are recommended. Apple juice and sodas are good; citrus juices are not. Neither are alcoholic beverages. For more severe cases, sports drinks like Gatorade or Powerade may be more useful because they replace sugars and electrolytes. (While these drinks are not completely clear, they are translucent—like sodas—and are therefore okay to drink. However, drinking too much Gatorade or Powerade can cause diarrhea.) Outside the United States, you may also be able to find electrolyte powder, to be dissolved in safe water and drunk at intervals until the diarrhea abates. In very severe cases, rehydration solutions such as Pedialyte may be necessary, especially for children with diarrhea.

Drink plenty of fluids even if you don't feel thirsty—at least six to eight ounces every two hours. It's fine to sweeten your drinks with a spoonful of sugar, too, because glucose (in sucrose, or table sugar) aids the absorption of water by the gut. That's why regular sodas may help, but diet sodas should be avoided.

Products such as Kaolin and pectin (Kaopectate) will give the stool a firmer consistency. Medications that work to slow the bowel include paragoric and opiates—available by prescription only—as well as diphenoxylate (Lomotil) and loperamide (Imodium). These provide quick but temporary relief by reducing muscle spasms in the gastrointestinal tract. They should be used only for a few days, however, as both are synthetic opiates and have some addicting potential—and in any event, longer-lasting illnesses should be evaluated by a doctor. Pepto Bismol is also a popular remedy that seems to work pretty well, though it does turn the stool and tongue black, so don't be alarmed when that happens.

Be aware, however, that using these remedies for symptomatic relief might not be the best course of action, particularly when bacteria are the cause. While they may make you more comfortable, they suppress the diarrhea that helps bring the offending bacteria out of your system. If you slow down the process, the bugs are going to linger longer.

After the first twenty-four hours of a serious bout with diarrhea, a little food is probably okay. It may be best, however, to try to go without food for as long as possible. Still, if you are really hungry, try going on a BRAT diet—bananas, rice, applesauce, and white toast. The bananas work to bind the stool together, slowing the movement a little, while the rice, applesauce, and dry toast are low-fiber foods and hence easily digested. Some sort of porridge—Cream of Rice, for example—is also good. Whatever you do, abandon the fiber. Now is not the time for a bran muffin or a slice of whole-wheat toast to start speeding things through your gastrointestinal tract.

Some people say they do well eating yogurt, believing its active cultures contain "good" bacteria that your gut is in short supply of since it became poisoned by the "bad" bacteria that caused the diarrhea in the first place. Some say yogurt is particularly effective for diarrhea caused by antibiotics. Others, however, say all dairy products should be avoided in all instances. You'll have to see what works for you.

Herbs such as chamomile, ginger, and cayenne pepper capsules are also touted by some who are inclined to such remedies. Their effectiveness hasn't been studied scientifically. Other herbal remedies that some swear by include garlic tea and ginger. Garlic is an antimicrobial, meaning it kills bacteria—or at least keeps them from multiplying. Ginger is said to soothe the gastrointestinal tract.

## When to Call the Doctor

If you have been affected with diarrhea and there has been no improvement after three or four days, it is probably time to see your doctor.

You should call the doctor right away, though, if there is blood in the stool or if the stool looks like black tar. The same goes for a fever over 101°F, severe abdominal or rectal pain, and severe dehydration as evidenced by dry mouth, wrinkled skin, or the fact that urination has stopped. Weight loss of more than five pounds in just a few days is also a reason to see a doctor. Moreover, chronic diarrhea may be an indication of irritable bowel syndrome (IBS), and your doctor may want to evaluate you for that condition *(see* Chapter 4, Irritable Bowel Syndrome).

There are forms of chronic diarrhea that have nothing to do with food but are the result of fluids secreted by the intestine. These are called secretory diarrheas and may be caused by undetected tumors, sometimes in the pancreas, that release hidden chemical messengers that tell the bowel to release large amounts of liquid. These tumors are difficult to diagnose, but can be identified by a series of blood and urine tests.

A problem called malabsorption, which occurs when the intestines fail to properly digest food or absorb the products of digestion, can also produce loose or soft stools that often are bulky, oily, and foul-smelling, but not necessarily diarrhea. There are a number of possible causes of malabsorption, rang-ing from vitamin $B_{12}$ deficiency, celiac disease, Whipple's disease, and eosinophilic gastroenteritis to kidney, liver, gallbladder, or pancreas malfunction. The cause of malabsorption may be challenging to diagnose, but can be identified via a series of blood and stool tests and other studies, such as biopsy of the lining of the small intestine via an endoscope.

# 8

# Excessive Gas

*To discover some drug, wholesome and not disagreeable, to be mixed*
*without common food, or sauces, that shall render the natural*
*discharges of wind from our bodies not only inoffensive,*
*but agreeable as perfumes . . .*
—Benjamin Franklin

A gurgling stomach, an unexpected belch, or, heaven forbid, a sudden blast from the anus—what is more humiliating than having gas declare itself in public? No matter that gas affects every member of the human race. When it occurs in a public setting, it's enough to make us want to run and hide. In ancient Rome, passing gas in a public place was actually illegal.

Fortunately, passing wind is not illegal these days. Now, we joke about it. We have funny, even impolite, words to describe it. But excessive gas—manifested in flatulence or belching or both—is no laughing matter for many people. In fact, while most people are not quick to run to the doctor complaining of gas, many actually believe themselves to have too much of it. And a million doctors' visits a year for the complaint suggest that, for many, excessive gas is more than just a nuisance.

Aside from causing embarrassment, too much gas can result in considerable pain, bloating, and discomfort, symptoms that may appear on their own or in conjunction with functional dyspepsia (FD) or irritable bowel syndrome (IBS). Very often, you may feel as if a balloon has been inflated inside your stomach. You feel distended, your clothes feel too tight, and it just gets worse as the day wears on. Sometimes, you may even hear and feel air and liquid swirling around inside.

Millions of dollars are spent each year on mostly useless remedies for gas. Many victims blame their symptoms on foods they love. Sometimes they are right, sometimes not. And doctors may not take complaints about gas seriously, as many have not studied the problem and don't know what to do about it.

Nevertheless, there are things that can be done, remedies that work. But in any case, other than offending our social sensibilities and perhaps causing some physical discomfort, gas causes no lasting harm to either our bowels or our bodies. That said, a little understanding of the problem can go a long way toward making it manageable.

## Where Does Gas Come From?

There are only two ways for gas to originate. Either you swallow it—aerophagia—or it is manufactured in the gut. It's a natural occurrence: everyone produces gas, and everyone expels it.

*Aerophagia* Upper gastrointestinal gas that erupts from the mouth as belches or burps comes from swallowed air that forces itself back up. In his book, *Gut Reactions,* Dr. W. Grant Thompson recounts the story of a young Frenchman who practiced the art of chronic belching in a bid to avoid being conscripted into Napoleon's army. This incident seems to be the first actual definitive description of aerophagia, but it certainly goes back long before that. Actually, there are two kinds of belching. One is a fairly innocuous condition that stops on its own about an hour after eating and is caused by air swallowed while eating. The other is more chronic and is caused by constant air swallowing—a nervous habit most people don't even know they have.

*Flatus* Gas that escapes from the rectum is mostly a by-product of the fermentation of undigested food and other bacterial action in the colon. This gas contains carbon dioxide, hydrogen, and, in some people, methane. Tiny amounts of volatile chemicals produced by bacterial metabolism of residual fats and proteins are responsible for the distinctive foul odor of flatus. While most of this gas is produced in the gut, a tiny bit of it may be swallowed air (which contains oxygen and nitrogen) that has made its way down to the lower gastrointestinal tract as well as some gas that has diffused from the bloodstream into the gut.

## A Gas Primer

The minute we begin breathing as a newborn, we begin sucking in air and producing gas. The air we all breathe is made up primarily of nitrogen ($N_2$) and oxygen ($O_2$), the gas we need to sustain life. When air is swallowed, it enters the gastrointestinal tract. As it moves along, the makeup of its component gases changes, as oxygen may dissolve in the blood while nitrogen is added from the blood. In addition to the oxygen and nitrogen breathed in, another gas in the intestine is carbon dioxide ($CO_2$). It can also be breathed in, but it is found in the duodenum as the result of a chemical reaction of bicarbonate ($HCO_3$) (secreted by the pancreas and by the cells lining the duodenum) with the acid from the stomach. Another source of gas is the colon, where hydrogen ($H_2$) as well as carbon dioxide ($CO_2$) is released when carbohydrates (sugars and starches) that haven't been absorbed through digestion undergo bacterial fermentation.

This fermentation process produces foul-smelling gases as local bacteria consume undigested foods that have not been absorbed by the small bowel and have made their way into the colon. These foods are mostly carbohydrates, sugars, and fats, with the carbohydrates found in such high-fiber foods as beans, broccoli, cauliflower, and brussels sprouts being the worst culprits. These foods, when acted on by colon bacteria, release gases such as methane ($CH_4$) and hydrogen sulfate, which smells like rotten eggs. Interestingly, the worst odor is related to strong-smelling sulfurs that make up just 1 percent of flatus.

Among lactose-intolerant people (those who are deficient in lactase, the enzyme in the intestinal mucosa needed to digest the milk sugar lactose), high levels of hydrogen also occur. In addition to its presence in flatus, hydrogen may be detectable in our breath, especially after a meal rich in carbohydrates.

Methane ($CH_4$) may be detected in about one-third of adults as well. Like hydrogen, it is produced by the metabolic action of bacteria, in this case specifically an organism called *Methanobrevibacter smithii,* which is capable of synthesizing methane from hydrogen and carbon dioxide. Oddly, methane is produced only in the left colon. People with colon diverticula, or small, fingerlike sacs that protrude from the colon's inner lining (*see* Chapter 5, Diseases with Symptoms Similar to Irritable Bowel Syndrome), tend to produce methane more than other people. It is possible that the diverticular pouches serve as pockets in which *M. smithii* can take advantage of passing hydrogen. Perhaps not coincidentally, both methane production and diverticula increase with age. Studies show that Americans and Europeans are more likely to produce methane than are Asians, possibly because of differences in diet. Women also produce more methane than men.

Most carbon dioxide ($CO_2$) production in the gut is the result of bacterial fermentation of unabsorbed sugars and starches in the colon. Eating beans will substantially increase carbon dioxide production, as will taking sodium bicarbonate for heartburn. Hence, it makes little sense to use bicarbonate-containing seltzers for gas.

## Where and How Gas Escapes

You hardly notice gas when it enters your digestive system, but while it is there, its pain can be intense. As for its escape, well, we've all created powerful gaseous emissions that we've feared probably could be heard all the way across town.

### Belching

Etiquette with regard to belching seems to depend on historical moment or the place on the planet where the oral gaseous escape occurs. In the England of King Henry VIII, for example, a loud belch after dinner was quite acceptable, and in China around the turn of the twentieth century, a sonorous belch was not only done for the comfort of the diner, but also to show the host that the guest's stomach was indeed full and that the dinner was a success. Additionally, there was for many years in Texas an annual belching contest. And even today, in barrooms across the world, releasing a boisterous belch is a rude but macho sign of beer-guzzling prowess. But be that as it may, in most places these days, belching is frowned upon as a gross violation of good manners and taste.

Technically called eructation, belching occurs when the

upper esophageal spincter relaxes and lets swallowed, pressurized gas escape from the mouth. It often happens in the course of eating a meal: you swallow air, which causes the stomach to distend; the lower esophageal sphincter (LES) relaxes, allowing the air to reflux into the esophagus; and then the upper sphincter lets down its guard—and you can hear the result across the room.

Despite the social taboo against belching, the release of gas from the stomach has its purpose: if the gas doesn't escape, it may cause severe pain by stretching nerve endings in the esophageal wall. Of course, some can hold gas more easily than others, and for most people, belching is involuntary. Some people can tolerate gas more easily than others, some simply belch more often than most. A study has found that healthy young people belch an average of eleven times in twenty hours, excluding mealtimes. Some people, though belch more and can even belch on demand—we all have known adolescents with the ability to belch out whole tunes whenever and wherever they wanted. This talent relies on the ability to swallow air in large enough amounts to burp on cue.

Belching may be caused by foods eaten or by aerophagia. Foods that can increase the urge to let out a belch or burp include onions, garlic, tomatoes, chocolate, and mints. All of them can reduce LES muscle tone and increase the likelihood of belching.

Aerophagia, or the swallowing of air, can be influenced by factors other than eating and drinking. Some people swallow air and belch, for instance, to temporarily relieve abdominal discomfort. This action, however, may only result in the creation of a disgusting habit with no real long-term relief being obtained. Others belch often when under emotional duress, or when they lie down on their bellies or sit upright after a meal. Children who suck their thumbs, people who chew gum, and people who smoke—particularly those who smoke pipes—generally swallow more air than others. People who wear dentures or who suffer from postnasal drip or dry mouth tend to swallow more air than others, too.

## Pain and Bloating

People who suffer from bloating and painful abdominal distension feel like they are literally full of gas. If only they could get rid of it, they believe, the pain and feelings of bloatedness would go away. While those with gas may *feel* as if they are going to explode, they often don't have any more gas than the next person. Sometimes, however, they do: In a recent study by Akinari Koide and colleagues from Chiba University School of Medicine in Japan, X rays did show increased gas in patients suffering from bloating. However, this study included only persons with IBS.

In the 1930s, Walter Alvarez, a doctor and writer affiliated with the Mayo Clinic, conducted an experiment on himself to figure out why he was feeling so much gas-related pain and bloating. To locate the gas pockets he thought must have been causing his discomfort, Alvarez X-rayed his abdomen each day, whether he felt gas symptoms or not. He was surprised to find out that the amount of air seen was the same each day, regardless of whether he felt gassy and bloated or just fine. Researchers later measured the amount of air in a normal bowel and found the average to be about six ounces—no more nor less than so-perceived gassy bowels.

The problem, it turns out, is primarily one of sensitivity. People who complain of pain and bloating actually have, if not the same volume of gas as anyone else, then just a little bit more, but it affects them disproportionately more because they are more sensitive. When researchers pumped the same amount of gas into their intestines, the patients who complained of gas and bloating reported considerable pain, while those who had not come in complaining of any such symptoms still felt fine. Sensitivity, though, may not have been wholly to blame: the people with chronic gas pain also exhibited impaired peristalsis and significant reflux of gas from the small intestine into the stomach.

These findings have led investigators to suspect that gas discomfort, like irritable bowel syndrome and functional dyspepsia, is to some extent a problem of perception. People with these conditions may just be more sensitive to stomach and bowel stimuli than the average person. In fact, vague complaints of gassiness are often a symptom of irritable bowel syndrome. That said, pain and bloating is still a gas problem to these people. It's just not a problem of excessive gas.

In addition to being overly sensitive to gas, these people probably overreact to liquids too. That's because instead of pushing everything forward, their intestines twitch and spasm, often moving their contents the wrong way. When forward-moving food meets food moving the other way, the bowel may swell and feel bloated.

Usually, although a sudden buildup of gas is benign, the pain it produces can cause a scare. Severe distension of the stomach, occurring spontaneously or immediately following a meal, is called magenblase (literally, "stomach bubble") and can be identified by X rays. This condition, often accompanied by hiccups, may be mistaken for heart or gallbladder pain.

Similarly disturbing is the splenic flexure syndrome, a painful spasm in the left upper colon, just below the rib cage, that is produced by collections of trapped gas. Dubbed pseudoangina by some experts, it may mimic cardiac pain and cause a real scare. It has no relation to exercise, as does true angina, however. Pseudoangina's localized trappings of gas may be related to irritable bowel syndrome.

Less frightening but more embarrassing is borborygmi, a phenomenon that is characterized by audible gurglings and rumblings emanating from the abdomen: These sounds are created by peristalsis. While the person experiencing them may believe the noise is so loud as to be heard in the next county, the sounds are actually loudest to the person who is producing them. Such a person, if shy, may feel extremely embarrassed even though the sounds go unnoticed by anyone else.

Bloating itself is almost never a symptom of anything serious, but it may accompany other more ominous problems such as peptic ulcers, bowel cancer, Crohn's disease, endometriosis, and ovarian cancer. Excessive gas and bloating may also accompany celiac disease, an intestinal malabsorption condition triggered by gluten, a protein found in wheat, barley, and rye. In celiac disease, as well as in chronic pancreatitis or lactose intolerance, nutrients that should be absorbed by the small intestine but aren't become fermented in the colon.

All in all, while everyday gassiness is usually nothing to worry about, any new and unusually severe onset should be checked out to distinguish a harmless case of gas from one that may be an indication of another, more serious problem.

### Flatulence

Gas escaping from the far end of the gastrointestinal tract—we call it passing gas, breaking wind, or farting—may be natural, but nowhere is it socially acceptable. There are no sanctioned contests that we know of, no places where a blast from the rectum is considered a compliment to the host. No, flatus is looked upon as a curse to respectability and is one of those deeds that is better done in private.

The average human intestine normally holds from 100 to 200 milliliters of gas, but researchers have found that over a twenty-four-hour period, production of flatus averages 2 liters. Normal individuals emit from 50 to 500 milliliters of gas fourteen times a day, with the upper range of normal in healthy young men reaching twenty-five emissions a day.

Fortunately, the mucosa of the upper anus has sensors that can distinguish flatus from feces. If not, the world would undoubtedly be a much worse place.

---

Flatulence is a normal part of the human condition. Great writers, scientists, and statesmen, in fact, have even written about it.

As far back as the fifth century B.C., one of the Greek playwright Aristophanes' characters groused, "My wind is not frankincense."

"It is universally well known That in digesting our common Food, there is created or produced in the Bowels of human creatures, a great quantity of wind," wrote Benjamin Franklin.

---

All this gas originates in the intestine, and its quantity and composition depend largely on what foods we eat. Studies using hydrogen breath-testing have found that up to one-fifth of the complex carbohydrates eaten by average, healthy individuals is turned into gas *(see* box, Learning from Our Breath).

## LEARNING FROM OUR BREATH

Scientists can determine how well our body digests certain carbohydrates by performing a simple and inexpensive procedure called a hydrogen ($H_2$) breath test. First, a sample of exhaled air is collected by having the patient, who has fasted overnight, breathe through the mouth (clips are placed on the nose) into a bag. Then, the patient drinks one glass of either orange-flavored lactose or cola-flavored glucose, depending on which of these two sugars is suspected of inducing gas symptoms. A breath sample is taken immediately after this and subsequently every half hour for three more hours. These samples are analyzed for hydrogen content to determine whether the patient is able to properly absorb lactose or glucose, or whether there is an overgrowth of bacteria. Lactose, or milk sugar, and glucose are normally absorbed in the small intestine but will be broken down by bacteria if present. Hydrogen is the by-product released when carbohydrates are attacked by intestinal bacteria in the intestine (when bacterial overgrowth is present) or the cecum (when the carbohydrate is not absorbed in the small intestine). This hydrogen is quickly absorbed and excreted in the breath. Hence, elevated levels of hydrogen in the breath sample is an indication of malabsorption of lactose or glucose or of bacterial overgrowth.

Special instruments measure $H_2$ in the breath through a process called gas chromatography. To judge carbohydrate malabsorption, $H_2$ concentrations in the interval samples are compared with the breath sample that was taken prior to the test. For example, a person unable to absorb lactose typically will show an increase in breath hydrogen of at least ten parts per million above the baseline sample after ingesting milk.

Elevated hydrogen breath levels that appear after fasting may also indicate a slowing of intestinal motor activity or an overgrowth of bacteria within the small intestine.

---

Throughout history, certain foods have been notorious for producing gas. Beans, of course, are the most famous. Beans contain the complex carbohydrates stachyose and raffinose, neither of which the intestine can absorb but both of which the bacteria in the colon love. The bean-gas problem is most serious in people who switch from a low-fiber diet to one rich in beans and other high-fiber foods. Their digestive tracts simply are not prepared with enough of the enzymes needed to digest bean sugars, so these sugars pass undigested into the lower intestine—where the bacteria get hold of them, metabolize them, and generate gas. If people eat beans on a regular basis, the problem usually lessens, because as the body adjusts to the new bean-rich diet, it begins to produce the enzymes it needs.

Other known gas producers include vegetables such as broccoli, peas, brussels spouts, cucumbers, and cauliflower; fruits such as apples, melons, grapes, raisins, and bananas; sorbitol, an artificial sweetener found in diet foods; and fructose, a sweetener derived from fruits and vegetables. Certain other foods and beverages, including carbonated drinks, souffles, and whipped desserts, are also notorious for producing flatus because they introduce air into the gastrointestinal tract (see box, Foods That May Cause Gas).

## FOODS THAT MAY CAUSE GAS

There is a great variation among the foods that can cause gas in different people. Some of the more common offenders are listed here:

| | |
|---|---|
| Apples | Grapes |
| Bananas | Milk and other dairy products |
| Beans, peas, and lentils | Nuts |
| Broccoli | Oats and other high-fiber foods |
| Brussels sprouts | Onions |
| Cabbage | Raisins |
| Carbonated beverages | Sorbitol |
| Cauliflower | Turnips |
| Corn | Wine |
| Cucumbers | |

Gas can also result from specific dietary factors and intolerances. People who are lactose intolerant, for instance, often describe distressing flatulence if they consume milk products. For them, just two grams of lactose in the colon can produce up to 1,400 milliliters of hydrogen—more than twice the amount of gas the average person expels in a day. One lactase-deficient person, after drinking just two pints of milk, claimed to have passed gas 141 times—and submitted the statistic to the *Guinness Book of World Records*. People with celiac disease, who can't digest proteins in gluten, may experience a similar problem with flatulence when they eat foods containing wheat, barley, or rye.

Other factors, such as disturbances in motility or metabolism, also influence how often and how much flatus is passed. For instance, people with slowed intestinal motility may produce more gas simply because bacteria have more time to work their magic on complex carbohydrates. Gas production may also increase when people take antibiotics, because such medications introduce changes in the types of bacteria in the colon, or when the acidity level in the colon and bowel decreases.

## Diagnosing Gas

The important thing for a doctor to consider when diagnosing a belching, bloating, or flatulence problem is whether it is occurring on its own or in conjunction with one or more of the various functional gastrointestinal disorders or a more serious gastrointestinal illness. Gassiness may be the patient's only complaint, or it could accompany a constellation of gut symptoms that may or may not include nausea, loss of appetite, foul breath, and a feeling of fullness prior to completing a meal.

Although the functional gastrointestinal disorders are not dangerous in and of themselves, many of their symptoms overlap, so determining which is at work, and which of a range of individual treatment programs may be helpful, is sometimes difficult. And, of course, many of these same symptoms may indicate the presence of a more serious illness, so it is critical that the physician consider all possibilities. While the doctor may be able to quickly determine that the problem is the result of eating too many beans or of swallowing too much air, he or she should be alert to problems that may suggest organic disease, such as weight loss or anemia. In most cases, evaluating complaints of gassiness will not require extensive diagnostic testing.

### History
The first thing your doctor will do if presented with a complaint of gassiness will be to take a complete medical history, with a special emphasis on what you have been eating. Questions may include any of the following:

- What foods do you usually eat?
- Have you eaten any different foods lately?
- Have you recently increased the fiber content of your diet?

The patient may be asked to keep a diary prior to the office visit to find out whether the symptoms are linked to the consumption of specific foods. And if upper-intestinal bloating and belching are the major problems, excessive air swallowing may be the culprit. The doctor will ask about such habits as gulping down meals, drinking carbonated beverages, sipping through a straw, chewing gum, smoking cigarettes, and using chewing tobacco.

Questions will also seek to determine if you have a problem with lactose intolerance:

- Does it occur after ingestion of milk products?
- Is it better after withdrawal of milk products?

And the doctor is likely to ask about specific foods, if you have tried to withdraw those foods from your diet, and what the results have been. He or she will also likely ask whether you have tried any home treatments and if they have been at all successful.

Anxiety and psychological problems that may contribute to air swallowing and predispose people to irritable bowel syndrome symptoms, including gas and cramping, will be another avenue of inquiry. Likewise, the physician will want to review what medications you may be taking, since some, especially theophylline and drugs that are encapsulated with a sorbitol filler, may induce gas and bloating.

## Physical Examination
The physical exam will not usually show much out of the ordinary, although bowel sounds may be easier to detect than

usual with a stethoscope placed on the abdomen. An abdomen distended with air can be detected by listening for a hollow sound when tapped. Organic causes of intestinal distension may include obstruction of the bowel or ulcerative colitis, and accompanying signs of these disorders, such as tenderness over the colon, bloody diarrhea, or blood and pus on rectal examination of the colon, may be evident on physical exam. Some conditions, such as gastric distension, can be identified with a simple abdominal X ray. A doctor might also want to run a lactose absorption test or hydrogen breath test if lactose intolerance is suspected.

Since the problem is most likely a functional one with no serious threat to the patient's health, many sufferers are probably going to feel greatly relieved when they are reassured that there is nothing wrong with them. Gas is part of life and, as long as burping and breaking wind are not done in a public setting, most patients will probably get along just fine.

## Treating Gaseous Complaints

While there are some advertised medicinal remedies for "problem" gas, the key to managing symptoms of gassiness is prevention. The goals are simple: minimize gas and keep bowel function regular. In most cases, these tasks can be accomplished by altering one's diet and adopting some simple habits.

### Belching

The obvious strategy is to keep from swallowing air. Altering eating habits is a good place to start. Avoiding carbonated drinks and whipped desserts—which trigger burping—is an easy fix to reduce upper-gastrointestinal gas. Some swear by including certain foods such as brown rice or barley broth in the diet; papaya and pineapple are also said to help—the juices in these fruits are said to soothe the stomach and keep it from becoming too bubbly. Whatever you eat, make sure to chew foods slowly, try to eat smaller meals, and avoid washing down food with liquids. And don't eat when you are anxious, upset, or overtired. Trading in loose dentures for snugger ones should cut down on air gulping while eating and at other times too.

Taking a brisk stroll after eating rather than taking a nap is a good idea for promoting gastric emptying and relieving the bloated feeling. Rocking in a rocking chair may also help. And when it is time to go to bed, try sleeping on your stomach or on the right side to aid in the escape of gas, which will help to alleviate fullness.

Other habit changes may prove helpful as well. Quitting smoking and laying off chewing gum can reduce aerophagia, and if you are a nonstop talker, try shutting up for a while.

Those who have a problem with sucking in air unconsciously and with chronic belching may be able to learn how to stop by watching themselves in the mirror. Biofeedback and hypnosis have also been tried by some, with mixed results.

Symptoms of pain and bloating may be helped by regular bowel function. Gradually adding fiber to the diet and using laxatives as needed can reduce constipation and speed up the transit of food through the system. Fiber, however, can increase gassiness, at least at first, so it must be added carefully, little by little.

There are a number of products advertised to reduce gas symptoms, and these can be an alternative too. Some are used alone and contain simethicone (Gas-X, Phazyme, Mylicon), or in conjunction with antacids. They are designed to break up large collections of gas bubbles, relieving symptoms, but their effectiveness is debatable.

If your small intestine is unable to properly digest and

break down the sugars that constitute carbohydrates, then the undigested carbs will travel into your colon, where resident bacteria will use them for fuel. This will result in gas and bloating. Sometimes this condition can be cured with certain types of oral antibiotics.

## Flatulence

This one is easy: quit eating the foods that are causing you all that gas. Restricting culpable foods—beans, fruits, and other complex carbohydrates, as well as the artificial sweetener sorbitol—may go a long way toward reducing, if not eliminating, the problem. Remember, though, that you don't want to eliminate all fruits and vegetables—just the real bad offenders. Fruits and vegetables, after all, are the basis of a healthy diet.

One possible way around the problem of food-induced flatulence is a product called Beano, which contains an enzyme, alpha-galactosidase, that helps the body to metabolize difficult-to-digest complex carbohydrates. The maker recommends sprinkling about five drops of the liquid on top of cooked beans or other gas-producing foods just before you take the first bite, or chewing Beano tablets just before eating.

Some beans are worse than others, too, so look for ones that are mild if you want to keep beans in your diet. Lima beans and lentils are considered the easiest beans to digest. Then, all beans are less likely to cause problems if you soak them for four to five hours overnight, then drain, rinse, and cook them in water. Canned beans may also be easier to digest, since they are usually well cooked.

There is no shortage of dietary steps that purportedly help alleviate the winds. For some, a drastic reduction in sugars in the diet and some cutbacks in starches (from potatoes and rice, for example) and wheat flour may help. Other people recommend eating foods in different combinations.

For instance, proteins and starches together may be a bad mix, as may be fruits along with vegetables. And still other people advise adding fresh papaya (which contains papain) and fresh pineapple (which contains bromelain) to the diet; papain and bromelain are digestive enzymes that may prove beneficial in reducing gas. Finally, brewing a tea with one or two teaspoons of anise or fennel seeds per cup of boiling water is an old folk remedy. Other supposed gas-relieving teas include those made with chamomile, ginger, and peppermint.

Activated charcoal, a tasteless black powder, absorbs gas and for some people works to cut down on gassiness, particularly after high-carbohydrate meals. In studies, charcoal capsules reduced the rise of breath hydrogen following ingestion of beans. But because they can interfere with the absorption of other medications and nutrients, charcoal capsules should be taken separately from meals and should not be used for long periods of time. Occasional use is not harmful, however, and there are no side effects. Antacids themselves may be tried, but evidence is that they may work best as a placebo. Preparations containing pancreatic enzymes (Phazyme) have also been tried, but evidence of efficacy is spotty.

Anticholinergics, drugs that block the nerves that stimulate the digestive tract, have also been tried with some success by people pursuing gas relief. However, these prescription drugs may carry with them a host of unpleasant side effects. Similarly, antidepressants and tranquilizers may work by calming the nerves or lessening anxiety, but these must be used carefully and only under a doctor's close supervision.

That said, gas, bloating, and flatulence are, have been, and always will be a part of life. It is unlikely that we will ever be able to eliminate them entirely.

# 9
# Food Allergies and Intolerances

The gastrointestinal symptoms produced by food allergies and intolerances and those caused by the various functional disorders of the intestinal tract are often the same.

For most people, heartburn, gas, nausea, and general stomach upset in the upper abdomen and diarrhea, cramps, and flatulence in the lower abdomen may result from such functional disorders as gastrointestinal reflux disease (GERD), irritable bowel syndrome (IBS), functional dyspepsia (FD), functional diarrhea, or functional constipation. For some people, however, these symptoms are caused instead by a food that, for some reason, simply doesn't agree with them. The food wasn't spoiled, unripe, teeming with bacteria, or crawling with parasites. No, the food was perfectly fine. It was the body's response to it that was the problem.

While there is disagreement over just how extensive they are, food allergies and intolerances are a legitimate problem. One recent report in a major national newspaper stated that 60 percent of the population has a food allergy of one kind or another. The U.S. government, meanwhile, pegs the figure at between 10 and 15 percent of the American population. Still, some allergy experts say that true food allergies are quite rare, particularly in adults, and place the number at closer to 1 to 2 percent of the general population and somewhere between 2 and 8 percent among children. Food intolerances, on the other hand, are considered much more common, according to the experts.

Sometimes, it is hard to know the difference. The most well-known food intolerance is lactose intolerance, or the inability to digest the sugars (lactose) in dairy products. It's been estimated that up to 70 percent of the world's population has some sort of problem with lactose, though it's minor for most. Another well-known food intolerance involves difficulties digesting wheat or substances that contain the wheat protein gluten. Lactose and wheat intolerance, which will be addressed later in this chapter, are the best known of food intolerances.

Food intolerances such as these differ from food allergies. Food intolerances, such as those to dairy products or wheat, may manifest themselves as a result of a direct chemical toxic effect every time a person eats a particular food. Food allergies, on the other hand, are hypersensitive and abnormal adverse reactions to food that involve the participation of the immune system. Even though the symptoms of the two can be similar, the immune system is not responsible for the symptoms of a food intolerance.

True food allergies are particularly difficult to diagnose, as allergies provoke reactions ranging from a swelling of the lips or tongue to an asthma attack to an episode of hives or eczema. As with intolerances, these symptoms usually occur each and every time the offending food is consumed. Genuine allergic reactions, however, occur within minutes of ingesting an offending food. Symptoms that arise more than an hour later most likely indicate an intolerance. Gastrointestinal symptoms, such as diarrhea, vomiting, abdominal pain, bloating, gas, and constipation, usually do not hit for an hour or more after eating the food in question, and therefore signal intolerances.

Foods frequently implicated in adverse reactions include eggs, milk, nuts, shellfish, strawberries, tomatoes, fruits, corn, yeast, meat, tea and coffee, chocolate, and fat—but that is only a partial list: there is probably someone, somewhere, who has difficulty with just about any food you can think of. Foods least likely to provoke an adverse reaction include lamb, rice, carrots, potatoes, lettuce, apples, and pears.

Many patients are quick to blame their gastrointestinal symptoms or even lip swelling and hives on food allergies. Most doctors, however, approach the subject of food allergies with caution because it can be difficult to prove that symptoms blamed on food allergies are really caused by food. Many of the perceived symptoms, such as nausea, vomiting, cramps, and diarrhea can have many causes. In addition, the diagnostic tests for food allergies are hard to interpret and unreliable. Intolerances—to dairy products or wheat, perhaps—are easier to pinpoint, because they are more common and easier to deal with. It is important to identify true food allergies because allergic reactions can be extremely dangerous. Food intolerances, on the other hand, are mostly just unpleasant.

## Adverse Reactions to Additives?

Additives that add color, flavor, or texture to foods can provoke adverse reactions as well. One such allergy that most people have heard of is to monosodium glutamate, or MSG, an additive used by many Chinese restaurants to enhance flavor. Reactions to this additive include gastric distress, headaches, and dizziness. If you routinely feel sick after eating restaurant Chinese food, next time out ask that your meal be prepared without MSG. That simple step may well solve the problem of "Chinese restaurant syndrome."

Sulfites, another common food additive and naturally occurring substances in many red wines, may also cause an adverse reaction in some people. Reactions vary, but abdominal pain is common. Usually, food labels list sulfites; prepared processed foods are most likely to contain them. Of all reaction-causing food additives, sulfites are the ones that most closely resemble true allergens.

FD&C Yellow No. 5, a food coloring, is commonly associated with adverse reactions and this is required to be listed on food labels. Aspartame, the artificial ingredient used in most diet sodas, also causes reactions in many people. While studies have shown that aspartame is not a true allergen, it nevertheless seems to cause an unpleasant reaction in many who consume it in diet soft drinks.

## How Allergic Reactions Work

Allergic reactions involve the human immune response in two ways. One is by stimulating the production of immunoglobulin E (IgE), an antibody that circulates through the blood. This tendency to produce IgE in reaction to certain normally benign foods is usually an inherited trait, and thus such food allergies run in families. The second immune response involves the mast cell, a leukocyte (white blood cell), that contains inflammatory mediators (chemicals which, when released, induce inflammation) such as histamine and serotonin and is particularly common in areas of the body where allergic reactions typically occur, such as the nose, throat, skin, and gastrointestinal tract.

IgE is found in tiny amounts in the body, but it packs a mighty punch. An immunoglobulin produced by plasma cells, IgE's main function seems to be to protect against invading parasites. It binds to allergens as well as to mast cells and triggers the mast cells to release substances that can cause inflammation. The surfaces of mast cells contain special receptors specifically for IgE binding, arranged such that when two adjacent mast-cell-linked IgE antibodies are in place, an allergen is drawn to both and attaches itself to both, cross-linking them. When a critical mass of IgEs become linked in this manner, the mast cell releases histamine and other inflammatory substances and the allergic cascade starts.

The process basically works like so: When the problem food is digested for the first time, it spurs the production of IgE, which then heads to the mast cells. There, the IgE binds to the mast cells' surfaces. The next time this food is consumed, it interacts with the IgE on the mast-cell surfaces and triggers those cells to release histamine, the chemical that causes the symptoms in question. Where the symptoms occur depends on where the mast cells release the histamine. If it is released in the gastrointestinal tract, for example, abdominal pain or diarrhea can be the result.

Food allergens—the food particles responsible for the allergic reaction—are proteins that are not broken down by cooking or during digestion in the stomach by acids or enzymes. When these substances survive, they can get into the gastrointestinal tract, bloodstream, and elsewhere, causing allergic reactions throughout the body.

The digestive process determines the timing and place of a food-allergy reaction. Some people may begin to feel symptoms—perhaps a swelling of the lips—as soon as offending food enters the mouth. As the food moves along to the stomach, abdominal symptoms may develop. By the time the food hits the bloodstream, other reactions, including a drop in blood pressure, may occur.

## Diagnosing Food Allergies

Symptoms such as the onset of swelling of the lips or tongue, hives, or asthma within minutes of ingesting a certain food are fairly clear evidence of an allergic reaction. The symptoms that come later, perhaps up to an hour later, however, are tricky to diagnose. These latter symptoms include those in the gastrointestinal tract. The doctor's job is to decide whether these symptoms stem from an intestinal disorder or an allergy. Once an intestinal disorder has been eliminated, the doctor can focus on whether the problem is the result of a food allergy.

Taking a family history will help. We know that these allergies tend to run in families, so if you and your family have a history of allergies, it may be that your intestinal problems result from a food allergy. Other history helps, too. The doctor will also want you to recall the times when you have had allergic episodes. Sometimes, food-allergy reactions are so dramatic that you'll never forget them. In the case of a gastrointestinal reaction, though, that's not usually the case: it may be hard to separate times when you've had diarrhea and cramping owing to a reaction to food from times when you've experienced food poisoning, the flu, or symptoms from another cause.

The doctor will probably ask you a number of questions. Among them:

- Did the reaction come on quickly after eating?
- Did you take an allergy treatment, such as an antihistamine, and did it help?
- Is this reaction associated with only one food?
- Did anyone else get sick?
- How much of the suspected food did you eat?
- How was this food prepared?
- Did you eat other foods at the time of the reaction?

The answers to these and similar questions may help the doctor in making a diagnosis. Often, however, more information is needed. That's when the doctor will order an elimination diet, which involves eliminating one food from your diet at a time. So, when a certain food is removed and symptoms disappear, a diagnosis can be made. Sometimes, such a diagnosis is not certain until the patient goes back and eats the food again—if the symptoms return, that is seen as diagnostic confirmation. This process can be long and tedious, and also may involve skin or blood tests to objectively measure allergic reactions to food. These tests, however, are considered controversial and not particularly effective.

The final method of testing—a "gold standard"—for food allergy is the double-blind food challenge. Various foods are placed in unmarked capsules and the patient is asked to swallow each, then see if a reaction occurs. Because the patient doesn't know what is in the capsules, there is not likely to be a psychological component skewing reactions.

## Treatment of Allergies

The best treatment of any food allergy is simply to eliminate the offending food from the diet. Once the food you are sensitive to has been identified, just don't eat it anymore. Of course, patients must be careful—it's important to read food labels because many allergy-producing foods such as peanuts, eggs, and milk turn up in places where one wouldn't necessarily expect to find them. Because so many children have peanut allergies, most products that include peanuts are clearly labeled nowadays; nuts, in fact, can produce reactions as severe as anaphylactic shock. If your food allergy causes you gastrointestinal distress but nothing more, you don't have to be quite so vigilant. You may suffer for a while, but you'll live.

Some people have tried antihistamines to prevent food

allergies, but such medications seem to work best, if they work at all, on hives and hay-fever symptoms. They don't seem to work for gastrointestinal symptoms, and, even if they do, they don't seem to work as an after-the-fact treatment. Another, somewhat controversial treatment involves putting a dilute solution of an offending food under the tongue about a half hour before the patient actually eats that food, in an attempt to neutralize the second, potentially more troublesome exposure to the food. Similar to homeopathy, this is called sublingual provocative challenge. Studies have shown, however, that this treatment is not effective. One more treatment calls for injections of small quantities of the food extracts to which the patient is allergic. The shots are given regularly for an extended period of time in the hope of desensitizing the patient to the allergen. This approach has not yet been proven effective.

## Food Intolerances

Most people who believe they suffer from food allergies actually have food intolerances. The most common of these are lactose intolerance and wheat intolerance; others include difficulty tolerating citrus fruits and spicy foods.

Human food intolerances vary widely and provoke diverse reactions. Some are to specific foods and produce specific responses; these may be based on the presence—or absence—of particular enzymes. For example, many Asians experience flushing (redness and hot feeling in the face) when they drink alcohol because they lack a key enzyme that metabolizes alcohol. Food intolerances may also result from chemical toxic effects; as in the case of rapid heartbeat after the consumption of caffeinated beverages. Citrus fruits and spicy foods often provoke symptoms in persons with peptic ulcers, and fatty foods may cause problems for people with a defect in intestinal digestion or absorption, like those with pancreatic insufficiency. For many people who have difficulty tolerating certain foods, however, there is no apparent identifiable explanation, and the mechanisms that initiate their gastrointestinal distress often remain a mystery.

In the cases of lactose and wheat intolerances, however, there is no mystery. In both cases, thirty minutes after consuming dairy or wheat products, the affected individual develops gas, diarrhea, bloating, cramps, or nausea. These symptoms occur not as a result of an allergic reaction, but instead due to a direct chemical toxic effect.

The problem of lactose intolerance is widespread, but is more prevalent in certain ethnic groups, including Jews, Africans and African Americans, Native Americans, and Asians. Those who are lactose intolerant cannot digest sufficient amounts of lactose, the primary sugar of milk, due to a shortage of the enzyme lactase. Normally produced by the cells lining the small intestine, lactase breaks down milk sugar into simpler forms that can then be absorbed by the bloodstream. If there is not enough lactase to break down all the lactose, unsplit lactose travels to the colon, where the colonic bacteria feed on it to produce gases and acids. For most people who have it, lactose intolerance is a condition that develops naturally over time, with symptoms associated not just with milk, but with any dairy products, including cheese, ice cream, butter, and some types of yogurt.

Of course, the problem is now widely known, and most people who have it know it. The best way to avoid the symptoms, of course, is to avoid dairy products, but for those who need them or love them, dairy products may still be able to be consumed if the lactase deficiency is partially corrected by adding a special enzyme preparation to dairy products. One of these products is called Lactaid, which is also available in a tablet form that can be taken before eating. Furthermore, there are now milks, yogurts, and ice creams that contain the enzyme and may be consumed by many people with lactose intolerance.

People with more mild forms of lactose intolerance may find that they can eat some dairy products if they do so with other foods. That's because one of the key factors in lactose intolerance is the rate at which the stomach empties. If you can slow the stomach's emptying, you may be able to reduce the symptoms. Yogurt may not cause as many problems as other dairy products, probably because it is fermented.

Unfortunately, try as one might to avoid lactose, many foods contain hidden milk or dairy products. Some breads, processed breakfast cereals, instant potatoes and soups, margarine, lunch meats, salad dressings, pancake mixes, and products containing whey—all often contain lactose. Kosher foods are a safe bet, however, since kosher laws mandate that nondairy foods cannot contain any milk products at all. And then there are alternatives to dairy, including soy or rice milk, available in health-food stores and many supermarkets.

If you are worried about not getting enough calcium without dairy products, try green leafy vegetables, sardines, and tofu, or supplements.

Another example of food intolerance is wheat intolerance, which is a reaction to the wheat protein gluten. This protein is found in wheat-containing flour, bread, cakes, and pastas, as well as in rye, oats, and barley. In afflicted people, ingesting gluten can cause such intestinal symptoms as bloating, gas, distension, and diarrhea. Like lactose intolerance, the problem arises from a defect in the body's enzyme system. Removing offending foods from the diet eliminates the problem.

Beware, though, of chalking up such symptoms to a simple gluten intolerance. Some of the same symptoms may be caused instead by celiac disease, a more complex, serious form of gluten intolerance. Also known as sprue, celiac sprue, or gluten enteropathy, celiac disease is an immunologic disorder in which gluten intolerance provokes actual changes in the intestine that result in malabsorption. In this disorder, part of the gluten molecule combines with anti-bodies in the small intestine, causing the normal brushlike lining of the intestine to flatten. The smooth surface thus produced is much less able to digest and absorb foods. Further exposure to gluten worsens the condition.

# 10

# Psychological Factors

*Man may inherit a sick, irritable nervous system, another may spoil a good one with bad habits or bad training, or a good one may be shocked out of action by the blows of circumstance.*
—Sir William Osler

It's no secret—emotions often find their outlet through the gut. Nerves, stress, emotional upsets, mental problems, and other psychological factors can wreak havoc with the gastrointestinal tract.

From the harmless butterflies we all experience before giving a talk or performing in front of an audience, which likely are just the result of anxiety, to the havoc wreaked on the gastrointestinal tracts of irritable bowel syndrome (IBS) patients, we know that psychological factors take their toll. Sometimes, it is nothing more than a stressful event such as an important exam or job interview that makes us feel queasy, nauseated, and jittery in the stomach. Other times, a buildup of stress over time can render the bowels spastic, leading to chronic nausea, vomiting, and diarrhea. Some say psychological factors are such powerful actors on the body that they can even lead to cancer. How and why does any of this occur? We're not 100 percent sure in fact. But we know that it does indeed happen.

We'll limit our discussion here to the effect that nerves, stresses, and emotions can have on our gastrointestinal tracts.

From what we've already discussed in Chapter 4, Irritable Bowel Syndrome, we know that IBS has no organic cause. This leads many to believe that it is caused by emotional conflict, stress, or some other psychological factor.

Stress, in fact, is known to stimulate colonic spasms in people with IBS. The colon, scientists know, is controlled partly by the nervous system, and studies have actually shown significantly higher stress levels in people with IBS compared to those who don't suffer from it. The connection is furthered by the fact that stress-reduction techniques have been shown to be effective in relaxing IBS symptoms.

Some believe IBS to be not only a reaction to stress but a psychiatric disorder in its own right. It is true that studies have found more psychiatric problems among patients with IBS than among other people; studies in England have shown that patients with IBS or dyspepsia were more likely than those with organic illnesses to have suffered a serious, personally threatening event in the prior year—such as the loss of a job, a divorce, or death in the family—or a stressful event in the past, such as physical or sexual abuse. Still, disagreement remains about any psychiatric basis for IBS: suffice it to say that there appears to be a significant psychological component to IBS, as well as to probably a whole host of other gastrointestinal symptoms.

# The Gut-Brain Connection

We know that the gut's automatic workings are actually governed by the enteric nervous system (ENS), or "gut brain," with its complex network of nerves, hormones, and neurotransmitters coordinating the job of digestion. An intricate nerve complex in the intestinal wall that communicates with the brain via the spinal cord, this nervous system is connected to the brain by the vagus nerve and by the sympathetic set of nerve fibers that emanate from the spinal cord. Although called the gut brain, the ENS is not a real brain in itself, since it likely does not store information. Instead, it is more like the spinal cord as it runs along the intestinal wall, sending messages back to the brain via the vagus nerve, which carries the feelings of nausea and distension. Sensations of pain, meanwhile, are carried through fibers that accompany the sympathetic nerves. The gut brain, then, is intimately intertwined with the brain in your head, meaning that the brain can sense strange goings on in the gut and alter the gut's behavior. At the same time, emotional disturbances can cause changes in the chemical activity of the brain, sending disturbing messages to the gastrointestinal tract. As a result, feelings in the brain can manifest themselves in the gut, highlighting the gut-brain connection (*see* box, Looking at Gut Reactions).

## LOOKING AT GUT REACTIONS

Early researchers relied on some remarkable yet basic observations to learn how the digestive tract responds to emotions. In 1833, William Beaumont, a U.S. Army surgeon, was given an inside view when Alexis St. Martin, a French-Canadian traveler, was accidentally shot in the stomach. The wound left a gastric fistula, or opening to the skin, that allowed Beaumont not only to observe the pumping, to-and-fro motion of the stomach, but also to see what happened when his patient expressed different emotions. In his journals, Beaumont recorded that when St. Martin showed fear, anger, or impatience, his stomach mucosa grew pale and produced less gastric juice. Studies have since found that powerful emotions evoke both increased and decreased stomach secretions, depending on the person and the situation.

In 1950, Thomas Almy and his associates conducted some rather bold experiments on medical-student volunteers to find out how emotions affect the colon. The researchers induced pain and stress by immersing students' hands in ice water and tightening the screws of a band secured around their heads. The subjects' colons responded by showing increased pressure and secretions.

In yet another experiment, a student agreed to let Almy view his sigmoid colon, the section of the lower colon near the rectum, using a sigmoidoscope. During the exam, someone else present mentioned cancer of the colon, and the startled student leaped to the conclusion that this was his diagnosis. The researchers watched the lining of his colon blush and contract rapidly, only to relax and regain its normal color when the student was reassured that he did not have cancer.

---

In 1909, Walter Cannon* found that when a cat is stressed, its entire gut, with the exception of its sigmoid colon, relaxes. In a human experiment in 1950, researchers measured colon pressure in a woman during a stressful interview. When she was saddened or tearful, colon pressure fell; when she was angry, colon pressure increased. In combat situations, primeval reflexes appear to take over, causing the sigmoid to contract to prevent involuntary evacuation of feces. Thomas Almy, a renowned gastroenterologist at Dartmouth Medical School who conducted several experiments on medical students (including one described in Looking at Gut Reactions box), decided after reviewing his data that in

* Cannon (1871–1945) was a physiologist and Harvard professor who was the first to use barium to visualize the GI tract.

patients with irritable bowel syndrome, the disorder is "not in the bowel but in the environment, and in the patient's attitude towards the environment."

Until fairly recently, the link between the emotional centers of the brain and the intestinal tract was thought to be exclusively via the connecting-nerve pathways. In fact, imaging studies of the brain are actually showing that functional gastrointestinal symptoms do not always necessarily result from disturbances in the bowel, but rather appear to emanate from dysregulation in neuroenteric pathways that alter pain thresholds, motility, and behavior. There is much evidence to implicate dysfunction in the nervous system as a significant factor in the symptoms of patients who meet the criteria for functional gastrointestinal disorders. These include the fact that stress is known to stimulate colonic spasms in people with IBS and that motility disturbances in such persons disappear during sleep. In addition, roughly half of the patients seen in gastroenterology clinics* with a functional gastrointestinal disorder also have depression or anxiety disorders, and data support the efficacy of antidepressants in the treatment of functional gastrointestinal disorders.

Even newer discoveries, however, have shown that the brain communicates with the gut in other ways. Science has learned that hormones, chemical messengers made up of chains of amino acids called peptides, are produced within the intestines, where they carry signals to make the muscles contract and valves open so that the organ works harmoniously. Advances in neuroscience have led to the discovery that these peptides are also manufactured and stored in the brain and its nerves, and that they can also signal other parts of the body. This allows the brain, in essence, to talk to the gut. Meanwhile, the gut and other organs make their own

* According to Dr. Douglas Drossman in "Psychosocial Aspects of the Functional Gastrointestinal Disorders" (*see* page 174).

hormones as well, sending them to the brain when necessary—in essence, talking back.

In animal models, a brain peptide called thyrotropin-releasing hormone (TRH) has been shown to increase the secretion of acid and pepsin in the stomach. This action, in turn, stimulates blood flow, muscle contraction, and gastric emptying—and, in experiments, produces ulcers. On the other side of the coin, other chemical messengers from the brain, including endorphins, may cut down on acid secretion and gastric emptying, thereby preventing ulcers from developing, at least under experimental conditions.

We know that the brain has a direct effect on the stomach, if only by the way that just thinking about eating can set off the stomach's appetite juices even before food gets there. But the action goes both ways: a diseased intestine can send signals to the brain as much as a troubled brain can send signals to the gut. A patient's depression, therefore, may be caused as much by a troubled intestine as his or her depression may be causing a distressed gut.

## Tension Myositis Syndrome

Dr. John Sarno, a back specialist at the New York University School of Medicine, has an interesting theory that states that many of the millions of cases of "bad backs" that plague Americans are stress- or emotion-related. His idea is that the mind, trying to repress hidden anger and rage over any number of emotional insults endured from childhood to the present, causes back pain as a way to deflect attention from those problems that are just too difficult for it to confront. Sarno calls this phenomenon tension myositis syndrome, or TMS.

In TMS, says Sarno, oxygen flow to the back muscles is reduced enough to cause extreme pain but no lasting harm.

The problem can be cured, he goes on to say, by patients themselves simply by recognizing the cause of the problem and "talking back" to the brain. It may sound too simple to be true, but thousands of his patients and many tens of thousands who have read his books claim that they've cured their chronic back pain this way.

In recent years, Sarno has expanded his thinking to include a host of other illnesses and medical conditions among those that he says are being caused by TMS. Among them are many ulcers and a number of gastrointestinal disorders, including many cases of heartburn, bowel irregularities, abdominal pain, cramps, excessive gas, and even constipation.

## The "Mind/Body" Movement

Certainly, the idea of "mind/body" medicine has caught on in America. The ideas of Norman Cousins, Deepak Chopra, Herbert Benson, Bernie Siegel, and Andrew Weil, among others, are all the rage. Their ideas all center on the same thing: the mind has the capacity to cure disease and improve health.

Conversely, of course, it also has the capacity to cause disease and injure health. As far back as 1950, Franz Alexander, in his book *Psychosomatic Medicine,* wrote: "the patient as a human being with worries, fears, hopes, and despairs, as an indivisible whole and not merely the bearer of organs—a diseased liver or stomach—is becoming the legitimate object of medical interest. A growing psychological orientation manifests itself among physicians."

Alexander believed that emotional upsets could result in such physical manifestations as stomach ulcers, for example. Yes, science in recent years has uncovered a link between *H. pylori* bacteria and ulcers, but it is also true that not every patient with an ulcer is infected with *H. pylori*. And plenty of people have *H. pylori* without ulcers. So something else may be playing a role; perhaps this "X factor" is the emotions.

More recently, Norman Cousins, an author and editor of *The Saturday Review* magazine in the 1960s and 1970s, cured a crippling, life-threatening disease of the connective tissue, ankylosing spondylitis, by watching funny movies and taking massive doses of vitamin C. In his book *Anatomy of an Illness,* he wrote of how he was told that his disease was incurable and how he reacted: "Since I didn't accept the verdict, I wasn't trapped in the cycle of fear, depression, and panic that frequently accompanies a supposedly incurable illness . . . deep down, I knew I had a good chance and relished the idea of bucking the odds."

In his quest, Cousins was at the forefront of the holistic-medicine movement. "Great medical teachers," he wrote, "have always impressed upon their students the need to make a careful assessment of everything that may interact in the cause and course of a disease." Hippocrates, continued Cousins, "was quintessentially holistic when he insisted that it is natural for the human body to heal itself."

Finally, predating Alexander and Cousins, some seventy years ago, Arthur Castiglioni, in his *A History of Medicine,* wrote that "a physician above all should keep in mind the welfare of the patient, his constantly changing state, not only in the visible signs of his illness but also in his state of mind, which must necessarily be an important factor in the success of the treatment."

## Psychosocial Aspects of the Functional Gastrointestinal Disorders

When it comes to looking at the specific functional gastrointestinal disorders that have been the prime subjects of this text, there is plenty of support among mainstream gastroenterology experts for the idea that psychosocial factors are important to these disorders in a variety of ways.

Dr. Douglas Drossman of the Division of Digestive Diseases at the University of North Carolina, for example, concluded in an important paper published in *Gut* in 1999 that there is clear support for psychotherapeutic treatments, especially on a long-term basis for all of these illnesses, not just irritable bowel syndrome. He also noted evidence for the benefit of antidepressants on these conditions as well.

Psychosocial factors, Drossman's paper said, influence the actual physiology of the gut as well as the modulation of symptoms, the course of illness, outcomes, and choice of therapy for gastrointestinal complaints. Still, the paper concluded that there is no one psychological abnormality that could be associated with these disorders. Rather, the problems appear to stem from various brain-gut interactions. "The varied influences of environmental stress, thought, and emotions on gut function help explain the variation in symptoms of patients with these disorders," Drossman stated.

These psychological factors combine with physiological factors to cause pain and other bowel symptoms, Drossman concluded, and there is little point in trying to separate the two: "Both are operative and the task is to determine the degree to which each contributes and is remediable."

Severe life stress, however, is a clear culprit, Drossman notes, pointing out that such traumas often are found to have occurred immediately before the onset of functional bowel disorders. Specifically, high rates of sexual and physical abuse have been found in patients with gastrointestinal disorders—as high as 56 percent of such patients. Also, those with irritable bowel syndrome frequently suffer from a number of psychiatric conditions that can include anxiety, depression, and hypochondria, according to Drossman.

Drawing from this, Drossman suggests that doctors evaluating patients for gastrointestinal distress also screen for anxiety and depression with a few simple questions such as whether the patient has been worrying, had difficulty relaxing or with sleep, felt low in energy, lost interest and confidence in him- or herself, and found him- or herself unable to concentrate.

If any of the answers are positive, further psychological evaluation is needed, Drossman says. And while treatment may be indicated, he acknowledges that some patients may balk, "noting that some patients are initially unwilling to accept a role for psychological factors in the illness." Those who agree to seek psychological counseling may be helped by psychotherapy, hypnotherapy, relaxation training, and antidepressant medications, Drossman concludes.

Further, Drossman's review of thirteen studies showed that in comparison to those who used conventional medical approaches, patients who tried such unconventional approaches had significant improvement of their bowel symptoms. Still, Drossman advises that further studies are necessary to determine which psychological treatment will work best with which type of patient.

Dr. Henry D. Janowitz, former chief of gastroenterology at Mt. Sinai School of Medicine in New York, is another specialist who believes that psychological and physiological factors alike come into play in the development and progression of functional gastrointestinal disorders. In his book *Indigestion*, Janowitz unequivocally states that "there is clearly a brain-gut connection [in gastrointestinal disorders]. Under normal conditions, this is a harmonious interaction which coordinates a complex and, as yet, poorly understood relationship. It is not difficult, therefore, to grasp that there may also arise at times, for a variety of reasons, a discoordination between brain and gut."

Janowitz continues with words that should resonate among all who suffer bowel afflictions: "For the time being, then, I believe we can conclude that emotional turmoil and daily stress do play a part, along with our customary eating habits, the use of alcohol, caffeine, and tobacco, and our general lifestyle, including the amount of exercise we obtain, in how our entire gastrointestinal tract 'feels' and its physical condition."

Clearly, the evidence shows there is a mind-body connection linking the brain and the many functional gastrointestinal disorders that plague millions of people around the world. Whether it is the mental or emotional factors that are causing the gut dysfunctions or the other way around is not known for sure; perhaps it is a combination of the two. But what is certain is that those with functional gastrointestinal disorders seem to do better when both components, body as well as mind, are acknowledged by health-care providers who make it a point to treat their patients in a holistic way. Emotions, illness, and wellness are inexplicably linked, and patients and those who treat them neglect this link at their peril.

# 11

# The Aging
# Gastrointestinal Tract

Few problems of advancing age are more common than those involving the gastrointestinal tract. From the mouth to the anus, the general rule is that if it can go wrong, it will go wrong.

It's a fact of life that all organ systems begin to lose function starting at around age thirty-five. Judging from listening to the elderly complain about their gastrointestinal woes, it seems that the organs of the gastrointestinal tract cause at least as many, if not more, problems than most others.

Heartburn woes plague the esophagus; pain and obstruction bother the small intestine; constipation, cramps, and diarrhea dog the large intestine. And, of course, even more serious woes can harm the liver, gallbladder, and pancreas.

Despite the complaints, however, experts say that the gastrointestinal tract actually stands up to the ravages of time at least as well as if not better than the other bodily systems, particularly the central nervous and cardiovascular systems, do. And plenty of people are living happy, full lives

with healthy digestive systems into their eighties and beyond. It's just that those systems are moving more slowly.

## How Aging Affects the Digestive System

Like all muscles, digestive muscles slow down with age.
They contract more slowly, take plenty of time relaxing, and
move their contents along at a more leisurely pace than in
their youth. For the most part, that's fine—unless you become impatient and take drastic measures to hurry things
along or develop a condition that needs a doctor's attention. The fact is that many of the aging gastrointestinal
system's failures can be prevented or corrected. Griping
about the ravages of age doesn't have to become a way of
life, though understanding them from top to bottom might
help.

### The Mouth

The changes begin at the top, in the mouth, where the number of taste buds begins to decline with age. The sensitivity
of those that remain decreases too. As a result, some older
folks lose interest in food and begin to lose weight and develop nutritional deficiencies. Losing teeth may also cause a
reduced interest in eating. Good dental care is important to
keep the teeth in shape so that eating doesn't become a
problem.

### The Esophagus

Swallowing can become difficult as we age. Such problems
are usually the result of neurological or muscular disorders.
The simple fact is that the muscles of the esophagus may
grow flabby in very old age, and, as a result, contract less vigorously around food after swallowing.

Acid reflux as well is often a problem in the elderly, the

consequence of the decline in esophageal contractions and less supple function of the lower esophageal sphincter (LES) muscle. So, expect more reflux with advancing age. However, since the aging esophagus may become less sensitive to acid over time, this reflux may not be experienced as heartburn. If it is so manifested, treatment using one of the many medicinal remedies suggested in Chapter 2 is recommended. Changing eating habits with age may also be a good idea.

Of course, any new onset of difficulty in swallowing should be evaluated by a doctor, as there is always a possibility that the problem may be related to cancer of the esophagus or to a motor disorder (achalasia, or the inability of the LES to relax in response to a swallow, probably caused by a malfunction of the nerves surrounding the esophagus), both of which become more common in the older years.

## The Stomach and Duodenum

The stomach continues to make acid as we age, but acid production in many older people declines due to years of carrying *H. pylori* infection in the stomach, which leads to chronic gastritis and atrophy of the stomach lining. While this does not usually interfere with digestion, it can lead to two disorders that are common in the elderly: vitamin $B_{12}$ deficiency, which can bring on anemia, and overgrowth of bacteria in the small intestine, which can result in malabsorption and problems with digestion. Both problems can be corrected with medication. And while the incidence of duodenal ulcers declines after middle age, gastric ulcers become more common. Unfortunately, so does stomach cancer.

## The Colon

Moving one's bowels may be the most frequent gastrointestinal challenge associated with aging, and the problem is usually the product of a poorly functioning or diseased large intestine. Problems with this organ can also result in diarrhea, hemorrhoids, cancer, and infection. In fact, one in every three senior citizens has one or more polyps in the colon. That's why colonoscopies are recommended on a regular basis after the age of fifty (*see* Chapter 5, Diseases with Symptoms Similar to Irritable Bowel Syndrome). Removal of such polyps removes the problem and doesn't give cancer a chance to start its ugly growth.

In general, less stool is passed after one reaches age sixty-five. This may owe in part to a change in diet toward softer foods, a diminished appetite, or less muscular activity and exercise. Constipation may also stem from neurological problems or be the effects of too many years of laxative use, though this is rare.

## Common Age-Related Gastrointestinal Complaints

All of the functional gastrointestinal disorders detailed in this book are common among the elderly.

### Irritable Bowel Syndrome
Though irritable bowel syndrome (IBS) is perhaps the most common chronic malady to persist from young adulthood into elder years, its onset is rare among the elderly. As in younger people, there is the danger that IBS symptoms may hide a more serious disorder, so efforts must be made to rule out organic causes, cancer in particular.

### Diarrhea
While diarrhea is common in older people, it is nevertheless important to distinguish it from fecal incontinence, a separate problem that is especially common and embarrassing in the elderly. Fecal incontinence is, basically, the inability

to control one's bowels. The most common cause is a fecal impaction, a condition resulting from chronic constipation in which the large bowel is chronically blocked by stool and stretched. The person loses awareness of regular signals to defecate; loose stools push to get out and accidents happen. The remedy may be to prevent constipation by changing one's diet or through bowel retraining. Diarrhea is more likely to be associated with fecal incontinence in the elderly than in the young. Other people develop incontinence as a result of stroke or injury.

## Constipation

Constipation affects one in three elderly people and is often brought on by bad habits—specifically, not enough fiber in the diet, not drinking enough fluids, too little exercise, the abuse of laxatives, the use of certain medications, and poor bathroom habits are usually to blame. Constipation is not, however, an automatic consequence of aging: pay attention to these aforementioned factors and the problem may well go away. Some older folks, however, dwell on their bowel movements to the exclusion of almost everything else. This is not good. Efforts should be made to get them interested in other things. If nothing else, it may take their minds off the problem. In any case, once they learn that it is not necessary to move one's bowels every day, they may decide that they no longer have a problem.

In some cases, however, constipation may be a signal of a more serious illness or may be mixed up with fecal impaction. Such problems, of course, must be ruled out, and help from a doctor is called for.

## Bloating and Gas

In the elderly, bloating and gas may be associated with constipation, fecal impaction, or some other process that blocks the intestine. In most cases, however, they stem from a person swallowing air or eating the wrong foods. Experimentation with the diet may solve the problem, although eliminating foods that may be causing the condition may not be a good idea if those foods are the ones supplying the person with the roughage needed for the digestive system to move things along.

## Belching

Usually the result of swallowing air, but possibly a side effect of loose-fitting dentures or the result of reflux, burping is a habit that may be broken with conscious effort. However, it may be harder to teach an old dog new tricks.

## You Can Live with It

The gastrointestinal complaints of the elderly must be taken seriously because they can cause a significant decline in the quality of life and because they may be signs of more serious disorders.

The most important thing to look for is whether any such complaint is a new one. If it is, there is more of a chance that it may signal something more serious. As a general rule, these complaints sneak up on us over time. Ones that develop quickly are often the most serious.

Fortunately, there are plenty of ways to treat gastrointestinal problems associated with aging. In most cases, the same remedies that work for younger folks will work for older folks. And there are many new and improved methods of diagnosing these problems and making sure that they are not the signs of a more serious condition. These days, there is very little of the gastrointestinal tract that can't be viewed or measured with one test or another. With endoscopy, ultrasound, computerized tomographic (CT) scans, X rays, blood tests, sigmoidoscopes, and colonoscopes, we can certainly find out if there is an organic cause for any gastrointestinal complaint. And fixing such problems is easier, too, with new surgical techniques such as laparoscopy.

They say that growing old isn't for the faint of heart. Perhaps, but most older folks are content, even happy, in spite of their gradually diminishing faculties. The key may be coming to terms with decline in functions, taking actions where possible, and shifting priorities as necessary.

The elderly are already the fastest growing age group in the United States, and with the baby boomers fast approaching senior-citizen status, all Americans are going to be hearing about the problems of old age more than ever. The good news is that with preventive attention—healthy diets, plenty of exercise, and the right medications—our golden years may be filled with pursuits other than complaining about bowel movements or the lack of them, heartburn, and gas.

# 12

# The Rome Criteria

As we have seen, chronic gastrointestinal disorders are not only quite common, but also cause an amazing amount of pain and suffering for millions of people worldwide. Gastroesophageal reflux disease (GERD), functional dyspepsia (FD), irritable bowel syndrome (IBS), and chronic diarrhea, constipation, and gas, as well as food allergies and intolerances, can wreak havoc on the gut. Complicating the problem is the fact that most of these disorders occur in the absence of any observed anatomical or physiological abnormalities. In other words, when doctors check, they can find nothing wrong. That's why they are termed "functional" disorders.

This unusual fact flies in the face of the usual medical diagnosis—and of science. Instead of a test or hard data to detect a problem, all doctors have to go by are the words of their patients. In most cases, patient testimony leads the doctor to seek evidence not of what the problem is, but what it is not. Myriad tests are run to exclude explanations for the symptoms and narrow down possibilities. In the end, all the patient is left with is an explanation of what he or she *does not* have, or a diagnosis based on exclusion.

In many cases, such patients have been told that the problem is "all in their head," that their illness is "psychosomatic." There's really nothing wrong with them, the thinking goes: Give 'em a sugar pill and a visit to the shrink.

But the symptoms are real, the patients say. And so is the pain.

The first mention of a functional gastrointestinal disorder in medical literature came 180 years ago. Yet even though such a prominent figure as Freud maintained that physical manifestations of symptoms may have nothing to do with anatomical changes, there was little mention of these types of disorders in the literature until about twenty-five years ago.

Over the past two decades, medicine has been paying more attention to the functional gastrointestinal disorders. As scientific interest in understanding them has grown, so has the interest among clinicians in treating patients with these problems. Even so, the initial enthusiasm and hope among researchers and clinicians that most of these symptoms might be explained as simply the result of motility dysfunction dried up quickly. It was just too simplistic. At the same time, the counterargument that these disorders are strictly psychological in nature has also been seriously challenged too.

Now, the accepted way of treating these disorders is based on what is known as the "biopsychosocial model"— that is to say, most experts in the field see the functional gastrointestinal disorders stemming from a combination of biological, psychological, and social origins. As a result, most doctors nowadays are not likely to dismiss such complaints without recommending a diagnosis and treatment plan. One tool they have in this regard is the Rome criteria.

In 1988, the world's leading gastroenterologists and others interested in gastrointestinal illnesses convened in Rome. There, they developed a system that enables doctors to evaluate bowel complaints and render a diagnosis. These diagnostic criteria were updated in 2000, after a four-year effort.

The so-called Rome criteria have generated controversy, to be sure, but they have also put some much-needed energy into the study of functional gastrointestinal disorders. Everyone involved in the field—gastroenterologists, primary-care doctors, epidemiologists, researchers, psychiatrists, psychologists, health-care insurers, and patients—has his or her own view on the matter.

Still, all debates aside, the Rome criteria are now accepted as the standard of care for gastrointestinal disorders. The criteria have given these disorders a profile, which helps doctors diagnose and evaluate, and patients know whether they have a legitimate organic illness.

## The Rome Criteria

### Irritable Bowel Syndrome
At least twelve weeks, which need not be consecutive, in the preceding twelve months, of abdominal discomfort or pain that has at least two of three of the following features:

- Relieved with defecation
- Onset associated with a change in frequency of stool
- Onset associated with a change in form (appearance) of stool

### Functional Abdominal Bloating
At least twelve weeks, which need not be consecutive, in the preceding twelve months, of:

- Feeling of abdominal fullness, bloating, or visible distension

☞ Insufficient criteria for a diagnosis or functional dyspepsia, IBS, or other functional disorder

## Functional Constipation

At least twelve weeks, which need not be consecutive, in the preceding twelve months, of two or more of the following:

☞ Straining in more than one-quarter of defecations
☞ Lumpy or hard stools in more than one-quarter of defecations
☞ Sensation of incomplete evacuation in more than one-quarter of defecations
☞ Sensation of anorectal obstruction or blockage in more than one-quarter of defecations
☞ Manual maneuvers to facilitate more than one-quarter of defecations
☞ Fewer than three defecations per week

## Functional Diarrhea

At least twelve weeks, which need not be consecutive, in the preceding twelve months, of:

☞ Liquid (mushy) or watery stools
☞ Present more than three-quarters of the time
☞ No abdominal pain

## Functional Abdominal Pain Syndrome

At least six months of:

☞ Continuous or nearly continuous abdominal pain
☞ No or only occasional relation of pain to physiological events (eating, defecation, or menses, for example)
☞ Some "loss of daily functioning"—that is, interference

with usual activities (going to work, caring for children, and the like)

☞ The pain is not feigned

☞ Insufficient criteria exists for other functional gastrointestinal disorders that would explain the abdominal pain

Some professionals continue to criticize the criteria, noting that they are not physiologically based, were determined by consensus of the experts rather than through clinical trials, and are subject to change over time. Those who agreed upon the diagnostic criteria concede that no physiological criteria have emerged, but nevertheless insist the symptom-based criteria have stood the test of time since they were first outlined in 1988. Furthermore, backers of the criteria say that they have proven their value in clinical trials and have reduced the costs of caring for patients by sparing them the need for undergoing many unneeded diagnostic tests.

Still, they accept that the criteria may change over time as more studies are conducted, just as the most recent publication of the criteria has included subtle changes from the 1988 version. The effort, they say, is aimed at "legitimizing the conditions for our patients."

For many patients, the effort has been much appreciated.

# 13

# Good Gut Hygiene: Some Concluding Thoughts

Chronic gastrointestinal distress is no trivial matter, and knowing that the problem is a functional disorder with no structural abnormality or cause only makes it more frustrating. Usually, there's no one thing you can do, no one pill to take or operation to undergo, that will make the problem go away.

Accordingly, dealing with a temperamental digestive tract is probably going to take a positive attitude, an understanding doctor, and a commonsense approach to treatment. Yes, your problems are real. But, no, they are not life-threatening. And they don't have to ruin your life.

While this book has focused on defining the functional gastrointestinal disorders—pinpointing what they are and what they are not—and has looked at various treatment options, sufferers should know that the most important thing they can do is to use good old common sense in seeking relief.

Spending one's life looking for a cure may turn out to be disappointing, but adopting healthy lifestyle changes can only help. Though many are outlined in the course of this book, such changes of habit are critical enough to be stressed again as we conclude our look at the problem of the sensitive gut.

Basic among these commonsense approaches is to take control of your diet. Eat a balanced diet that includes plenty of fiber. Eat smaller meals. Eliminate caffeine (especially coffee), tobacco, and alcohol consumption. And stay away from foods that seem to upset the stomach, and, especially, make sure the food you eat is safe. Pass on foods that appear to be unripe or spoiled. When traveling, drink only bottled water and skip street vendors. You'll cut down on your chances of picking up "traveler's diarrhea."

Try to avoid medications that cause trouble, and if conventional gastrointestinal medications don't work, try herbal or alternative remedies. Some of them have proven helpful and, in any case, they are unlikely to hurt. Still, discuss these strategies with your doctor.

Try to relax. If you can't do it on your own, get help with tapes, books, or videos on the subject. Or take a class on one of the world's many relaxation techniques if you can find one in your town. Stress is a leading cause of many gastrointestinal disorders and reducing it can help you not only find relief from your gut symptoms, but in many other ways too. Exercise is also a good tonic for the gut as well as for the mind. A regular exercise program under your doctor's supervision may be just the trick for turning that sensitive gut around—and it'll help your general physical and mental health to boot.

Don't forget: the gastrointestinal tract doesn't operate in a vacuum. Problems in other parts of the body, including the mind, can have repercussions on the gut. Live as healthy a lifestyle as possible, in body and mind.

Although you may find it necessary to consult a doctor at times, you may find that following these commonsense approaches to the gut and life makes those times less frequent.

# Appendix: Drugs Used to Treat Functional Gastrointestinal Disorders

Pregnant or nursing women should not take any of these drugs except on the specific advice of a physician.

# ANTACIDS

| Active Ingredient* | Brand Name | Use | Side Effects | Comments |
|---|---|---|---|---|
| alumina, aluminum carbonate, aluminum hydroxide | Amphojel, Basaljel, Gaviscon, Maalox, Mylanta | Relieve heartburn and functional dyspepsia pain and promote ulcer healing by neutralizing stomach acid | Constipation; excessive and prolonged doses may cause bone pain, feeling of discomfort, appetite loss, mood changes, muscle weakness | Side effects are more likely for people with kidney disease; aluminum-containing antacids are not advised for elderly people with bone disease or Alzheimer's disease; do not use within 3–4 hours of taking tetracycline-type antibiotics |
| calcium carbonate | Alka-Mints, Rolaids, Tums | | Chalky taste, constipation; excessive and prolonged doses may cause difficult, painful, or frequent urination, appetite loss, mood changes, muscle pain or twitching, nausea, restlessness, unpleasant taste | Side effects are more likely for people with kidney disease |
| magaldrate | Lowsium, Riopan | | Chalky taste; constipation; excessive and prolonged doses may cause bone pain, feeling of discomfort, appetite loss, difficult or painful urination, mood changes, muscle weakness, dizziness, irregular heartbeat | Magaldrate is a chemical combination of aluminum hydroxide and magnesium hydroxide; side effects are more likely for people with kidney disease; do not use within 3–4 hours of taking tetracycline-type antibiotics |

| magnesia, magnesium carbonate, magnesium hydroxide, magnesium trisilicate | Gaviscon, Gelusil, Maalox, Mylanta, Phillips' Milk of Magnesia | Chalky taste; excessive and prolonged doses may cause difficult or painful urination, dizziness, irregular heartbeat, loss of appetite, mood changes, muscle weakness | Side effects are more likely for people with kidney disease; do not use within 3–4 hours of taking tetracycline-type antibiotics |
| sodium bicarbonate | Alka-Seltzer, baking soda | Abdominal fullness, belching; excessive and prolonged doses may cause frequent urge to urinate, mood changes, muscle pain, nausea, restlessness | Not advisable for people on low-sodium diets; side effects are more likely for people with kidney disease |

* Most over-the-counter antacids contain at least two, and often more, of these active ingredients.

## ANTICHOLINERGICS / ANTISPASMODICS

| Generic Name | Brand Name | Use | Side Effects | Comments |
| --- | --- | --- | --- | --- |
| atropine with hyoscyamine and phenobarbital | Arco-Lase Plus | Relieve gastrointestinal cramps, spasms | Dry mouth, difficulty urinating or urinary retention, blurred vision, rapid heartbeat, increased ocular tension, headache, nervousness, drowsiness; antispasmodics that contain phenobarbital may cause sedation, drowsiness, or, rarely, agitation | Should not be used by people with glaucoma; a physician should be consulted about concurrent use because this drug blocks or boosts the actions of many other medications; phenobarbital may decrease the effect of anticoagulants and may be habit-forming |
| atropine with hyoscyamine, phenobarbital, and scopolamine | Donnatal | | | |
| dicyclomine | Bentyl | | | |
| hyoscyamine | Levsin | | | |

# ANTIDIARRHEAL AGENTS

| Generic Name | Brand Name | Use | Side Effects | Comments |
|---|---|---|---|---|
| diphenoxylate and atropine | Lomotil | Stop diarrhea by slowing down intestinal movement | Abdominal discomfort, constipation; less frequently may cause blurred vision, urinary discomfort, dry mouth or skin, rapid heartbeat, restlessness, warm, flushed skin | Drink plenty of fluids; may be habit-forming; not to be used with alcohol or other depressants |
| loperamide | Imodium, Imodium A-D | | Abdominal discomfort, constipation; rarely may cause drowsiness, dizziness, dry mouth, nausea, vomiting, rash | Drink plenty of fluids; should be used with caution by people with liver disease |

# HISTAMINE H$_2$ - RECEPTOR ANTAGONISTS

| Generic Name | Brand Name | Use | Side Effects | Comments |
|---|---|---|---|---|
| cimetidine | Tagamet | Relieve heartburn and functional dyspepsia pain and promote ulcer healing by decreasing amount of stomach acid produced | Rarely may cause diarrhea, constipation, dizziness, drowsiness, headache, irregular heartbeat, increased sweating, burning, itching, redness of skin, fever, confusion in ill or elderly people | May interfere with the absorption of some anticoagulants, antidepressants, and hypertension medications |
| famotidine | Pepcid | | | No serious drug interactions known |
| nizatidine | Axid | | | |
| ranitidine | Zantac | | | At high doses may interact with anticoagulants |

# MUCOSAL-COATING DRUG

| Generic Name | Brand Name | Use | Side Effects | Comments |
|---|---|---|---|---|
| sucralfate | Carafate | Promotes ulcer healing and protects against gastro-esophageal reflux damage by coating the stomach mucosa | Constipation; rarely may cause gastrointestinal upset, hives | A physician should be consulted about concurrent use because this drug may interfere with the actions of other medications |

# PROKINETIC AGENT

| Generic Name | Brand Name | Use | Side Effects | Comments |
|---|---|---|---|---|
| metoclopramide | Reglan | Treat gastro-esophageal reflux disease or constipation by accelerating gastric emptying and peristalsis | Diarrhea; less frequently may cause involuntary movement of limbs, restlessness, drowsiness | Adds to the effect of alcohol and other depressants; caution advised for patients with Type I diabetes or Parkinson's disease |

## PROTON-PUMP INHIBITORS

| Generic Name | Brand Name | Use | Side Effects | Comments |
|---|---|---|---|---|
| lansoprazole | Prevacid | Treat reflux esophagitis and promote peptic ulcer healing by suppressing secretion of stomach acid | Rarely may cause diarrhea, abdominal pain, nausea | May speed the elimination of theophylline |
| omeprazole | Prilosec | | Rarely may cause constipation, chest pain, headache, gas, rash, drowsiness | May prolong the effect of other prescription drugs, including diazepam, warfarin, and phenytoin |
| rabeprazole | Aciphex | | | |
| pantoprazole | Protonix | | | Also available as an IV formulation |
| esomeprazole | Nexium | | | |

## TRICYCLIC ANTIDEPRESSANTS

| Generic Name | Brand Name | Use | Side Effects | Comments |
|---|---|---|---|---|
| amitriptyline | Elavil, Endep | Relieve chronic abdominal pain | Dizziness, dry mouth, blurred vision, drowsiness, constipation, urinary retention, hypotension, cardiac arrhythmias | Should not be used with alcohol, other depressants, or immediately following a heart attack; side effects may be worse when cimetidine is used simultaneously; caution advised for patients with glaucoma |
| desipramine | Norpramin | | | |
| nortriptyline | Pamelor | | | |

# SELECTIVE-SEROTONIN-REUPTAKE INHIBITORS

| Generic Name | Brand Name | Use | Side Effects | Comments |
|---|---|---|---|---|
| fluoxetine | Prozac | Relieve chronic abdominal pain | Rash, headache, dizziness, insomnia, anxiety, drowsiness and fatigue, excessive sweating, nausea, diarrhea, bronchitis, weight loss; muscle, joint, and back pain; painful menstruation, sexual dysfunction, urinary-tract infection, chills | Data for effectiveness in functional bowel disorders are limited |
| paroxetine | Paxil | | Pain, bodily discomfort, hypertension, syncope (a sudden loss of strength), tachycardia (excessively rapid heartbeat), pruritis (intense itching), nausea and vomiting, weight gain and loss, central nervous system stimulation, depression, emotional instability, vertigo (a hallucination of movement), cough | |
| sertraline hydrochloride | Zoloft | | Upset stomach, trouble sleeping, diarrhea, dry mouth, sexual side effects, unusual drowsiness or fatigue, tremor, indigestion, increased sweating, increased irritability or anxiety, decreased appetite | |

# OTHER AGENTS

| Active Ingredient | Brand Name | Use | Side Effects | Comments |
|---|---|---|---|---|
| activated charcoal | Actidose-Aqua, Charcocaps, Insta-Char, Liqui-Char | Relieve intestinal gas | Black stools, abdominal pain | Efficacy is uncertain; do not take at the same time as other medications |
| bismuth subsalicylate | Pepto-Bismol | Relieves heartburn, indigestion, nausea, diarrhea; used with antibiotics to cure ulcers | Dark tongue, grayish-black stools; excessive doses may cause anxiety, constipation, dizziness | Avoid if allergic to aspirin or other salicylates |
| simethicone | Gas Relief, Gas-X, Mylanta Gas, Phazyme | Relieve pain from excess gas | No side effects known | Efficacy is uncertain |
| alpha-galactosidase | Beano | Reduces intestinal gas by breaking down undigestible carbohydrates into digestible sugars | | |

# Glossary

**AEROPHAGIA**  excessive air swallowing

**ALIMENTARY CANAL**  the gastrointestinal tract

**AMYLASE**  an enzyme secreted by the pancreas that helps digest carbohydrates

**ANGINA**  temporary insufficiency of blood flow through the coronary arteries, usually causing chest pain

**ANORECTAL DYSFUNCTION**  a contraction of the pelvic muscles and internal anal sphincter when they should relax

**ANUS**  the canal at the end of the digestive tract through which feces are expelled

**ASPARTAME**  artificial sweetener used in most diet soft drinks

**BARIUM STUDY**  sometimes called an upper GI series (if barium is taken by mouth) or a barium enema (if given from below), a series of X rays taken after barium sulfate is passed into the part of the tract that needs to be examined; allows the contours of the organ to be defined on the X-ray image

**BARRETT'S ESOPHAGUS**  an abnormality in which the squamous cells of the lower esophagus are replaced by cells resembling those in the stomach or small intestine; occasionally may transform into cancer

**BELCHING**  expelling gas suddenly from the stomach through the mouth

**BERNSTEIN TEST**  a procedure in which diluted hydrochoric acid is dripped into the esophagus to determine whether the acid causes chest pain

**BILE**  fluid secreted by the liver; helps break down fats in the small intestine

**BIOFEEDBACK**  the technique of making unconscious or involuntary bodily processes perceptible to the senses, sometimes by the use of an oscilloscope, in order to manipulate them by conscious mental control

**BOLUS**  a softened mass of chewed food ready to be swallowed

**BORBORYGMI**  gurgling, splashing sounds caused by the peristaltic movement of air and fluid within the intestine

**BOWEL**  another word for the intestines or gut

**CECUM**  the pouch at the beginning of the large intestine into which the ileum opens from one side and which is continuous with the colon

**CELIAC DISEASE (OR CELIAC SPRUE)**  a disease in which sensitivity to gluten, a protein found in wheat, rye, and barley, causes a malabsorption of nutrients; symptoms include diarrhea, weight loss, malnutrition, and anemia

**CHOLECYSTOKININ**  a hormone secreted by the mucosa of the upper small intestine; stimulates gallbladder contraction and pancreatic secretion

**CHYME**  a nearly liquid mass of partly digested food and secretions in the stomach and intestine

**COLON**  the large intestine, extending from the cecum to the rectum; it is divided into six parts: cecum; ascending, transverse, descending, and sigmoid colon; and rectum

**COLONIC INERTIA**  sluggish bowel

**COLONOSCOPY**  examination of the interior of the colon using a flexible viewing instrument

**COLOSTOMY**  *see* **OSTOMY**

**CROHN'S DISEASE**  a chronic inflammatory condition of the small or large intestine; associated with abdominal pain, diarrhea, fever, and weight loss

**DIAPHRAGM**  the flat layer of muscle separating the chest and abdomen; assists with breathing

**DIGESTIVE TRACT**   the group of hollow organs that forms a long, twisting tube extending from the mouth to the anus through which food is ingested, digested, and expelled

**DIVERTICULA**   finger-shaped sacs or pouchlike openings that protrude off the hollow tube of the colon; often develop with age

**DIVERTICULITIS**   condition in which diverticula become inflamed

**DUODENITIS**   inflammation of the duodenum

**DYSPEPSIA**   indigestion; characterized by upper-abdominal pain following meals; may be accompanied by bloating, nausea, vomiting, a sense of fullness, and general discomfort

**DYSPHAGIA**   difficulty swallowing

**ENDOSCOPY**   a diagnostic test that allows a physician to view the upper gastrointestinal tract via a flexible tube inserted down a patient's throat

**ENTERIC NERVOUS SYSTEM (ENS)**   a complex network of nerves in the gut wall that communicates with the brain

**EPITHELIUM**   the layer of surface cells that line the gut or skin

**ERUCTATION**   belching

**ERYTHEMA NODOSUM**   painful, red lumps beneath the skin, usually on the legs; associated with Crohn's disease or ulcerative colitis

**ERYTHROCYTE SEDIMENTATION RATE**   a screening test for inflammatory disease that measures the rate at which red blood cells sediment from a well-mixed sample of blood

**ESOPHAGEAL MANOMETRY**   a diagnostic test to measure the pressure and contractions of the peristaltic waves in the esophagus and the upper and lower esophageal sphincters

**ESOPHAGITIS**   inflammation of the esophagus

**ESOPHAGUS**   the tubular passageway from the pharynx to the stomach; also called the gullet

**FECAL IMPACTION**   hardened stool packs the intestine and rectum tightly, making evacuation impossible

**FECAL INCONTINENCE**   the inability to control one's bowels

**FECAL OCCULT BLOOD TEST**   a test to detect blood in the stool

**FLATUS**   gas expelled through the anus

**FOOD ALLERGENS** proteins that are not broken down by cooking or stomach acids and can cause allergic reactions throughout the body

**FRUCTOSE** a simple sugar found in corn syrup, honey, and many sweet fruits

**FUNCTIONAL GASTROINTESTINAL DISORDER** a gut ailment whose symptoms cannot be linked to any infection or structural abnormality

**FUNDOPLICATION** an antireflux surgical procedure that tightens the junction of the stomach and esophagus by wrapping a supportive cuff of stomach around the lower esophageal sphincter

**GASTRITIS** inflammation of the stomach

**GASTROESOPHAGEAL REFLUX DISEASE (GERD)** a condition in which food and acid flow back into the esophagus from the stomach, often causing heartburn and sometimes damaging the esophagus

**GASTROINTESTINAL TRACT** the digestive tract

**GI SERIES** a barium study also known as an upper GI series; a procedure in which orally ingested barium is used as a contrast medium for an X-ray examination of the esophagus, stomach, and upper intestine

**GULLET** the esophagus

**HEARTBURN** a burning pain behind the breastbone that often radiates to the neck; caused by reflux of food and acid into the esophagus

**HELICOBACTER PYLORI (H. PYLORI)** a spiral bacterium found at the surface of the stomach epithelium; a major cause of gastritis and peptic ulcer disease

**HIATAL HERNIA** a condition in which part of the stomach protrudes into the chest cavity through an opening in the diaphragm

**HYDROGEN BREATH TEST** a diagnostic test for carbohydrate malabsorption; measures the amount of hydrogen in samples of exhaled breath

**HYPERCALCEMIA** elevated levels of calcium in the blood

**ILEOSTOMY** *see* **OSTOMY**

**ILEUM**  the section of the small intestine running between the jejunum and the beginning of the large intestine

**IMMUNOGLOBULIN E (IgE)**  an antibody that is secreted by the intestine and that circulates in the blood

**INFLAMMATORY BOWEL DISEASE (IBD)**  a generic term for ulcerative colitis and Crohn's disease

**IRRITABLE BOWEL SYNDROME (IBS)**  a functional disorder of the gastrointestinal tract that typically involves a range or symptoms which might include intermittent abdominal pain and bloating accompanied by diarrhea, constipation, or alternating episodes of both

**JEJUNUM**  the section of the small intestine running between the duodenum and the ileum

**LACTASE**  an intestinal enzyme that breaks down lactose

**LACTOSE**  a sugar found in milk and dairy products

**LACTOSE INTOLERANCE**  the inability of the body to absorb lactose; provokes gastrointestinal distress

**LAPAROSCOPIC SURGERY**  minimally invasive surgery using tiny instruments and cameras inserted through small incisions

**LIPASE**  an enzyme secreted by the pancreas; helps digest fats

**LIVER**  the body's largest internal organ; secretes bile and is important in many metabolic functions, such as protein synthesis and drug absorption

**LOWER ESOPHAGEAL SPHINCTER (LES)**  an area of high pressure at the junction of the esophagus and stomach

**LUMEN**  the hollow part of a tubular organ

**LYMPHATIC SYSTEM**  a network of structures, including ducts and nodes, that carry lymph fluid from tissues to the bloodstream

**LYMPHOMA**  a malignant tumor of the lymphoid tissue

**MAGENBLASE SYNDROME**  "stomach bubble" syndrome; the accumulation of swallowed air in the stomach after a meal; usually occurs while lying down and causes extreme discomfort

**MALABSORPTION**  a condition arising when the small intestine fails to properly digest food or absorb the products of digestion; can result in weakness, diarrhea, cramps, and weight loss

**MAST CELL**  a cell in connective tissues and other places in the body—for example, the nose, throat, skin, and gastrointestinal tract—where allergic reactions typically occur; produces histamine

*METHANOBREVIBACTER SMITHII* bacteria in the intestine that help digestion and produce the gas methane as a by-product

**MOTILIN** a hormone of the gastrointestinal tract that stimulates intestinal motor activity

**MOTILITY** ability of the digestive tract to propel its contents

**MUCOSA** the inner lining of the gut

**MYOCARDIAL INFARCTION** heart attack

**OSTOMY** an operation in which the colon (colostomy) or ileum (ileostomy) empties through the skin of the abdominal wall

**PANCREAS** a digestive-enzyme secreting gland located behind the stomach

**PANCREATITIS** inflammation of the pancreas

**PARASYMPATHETIC NERVOUS SYSTEM** the part of the autonomic nervous system that contains chiefly cholinergic fibers (those activated by the neurotransmitter acetylcholine) and tends to induce secretion of fluid and chemicals from the intestine, increase the tone and contractility of smooth muscle, and cause the dilatation of blood vessels

**PEPSIN** a general name for several enzymes secreted by the stomach in order to break down protein

**PEPTIC ULCER** raw, craterlike break in the mucosal lining of the stomach or duodenum

**PEPTIDES** chains of amino acids that make up proteins; chemical messengers called hormones fall into this category

**PERISTALSIS** wavelike movement of intestinal muscles that propels food along the digestive tract

**PERITONITIS** inflammation of the membrane lining the abdominal cavity

**pH MONITORING** a diagnostic test used to detect reflux of acid from the stomach into the esophagus; an acid-sensing probe is inserted nasally and positioned above the lower esophageal sphincter

**PYLORIC SPHINCTER** a muscular valve at the lower end of the stomach that opens to the duodenum

**RECTUM** the final segment of the gastrointestinal tract, between the sigmoid colon and anus

**ROME CRITERIA** criteria generally agreed upon by experts to diagnose a functional gastrointestinal disorder

**SALIVARY GLAND** one of three pairs of glands that pour lubricating fluids, which contain digestive enzymes, into the mouth

**SECRETORY DIARRHEA** diarrhea caused by an excess of fluid secreted by the intestine

**SIGMOIDOSCOPY** internal examination of the rectum and sigmoid colon, performed via a tube inserted through the anus

**SLEEP APNEA** a condition in which breathing stops often—for brief moments—during sleep

**SMALL INTESTINE** a section of the digestive system that includes the duodenum, jejunum, and ileum and plays the major role in absorbing nutrients for the body

**SOMATIZATION** a condition in which psychological stresses manifest as physical complaints; the development of psychosomatic symptoms

**SORBITOL** a crystalline alcohol used as a sweetening agent

**SPLENIC FLEXURE SYNDROME** acute left–upper abdominal pain resulting from pockets of trapped gas

**SQUAMOUS CELL** flat, scaly epithelial, or outer lining, cell

**STOMACH** the hollow, saclike organ of the digestive system between the esophagus and duodenum; stores and grinds food, secretes acid and digestive juices that break down proteins, and pushes chyme into the small intestine

**STRICTURE** a scarred narrowing of the esophagus that can impede swallowing

**SYMPATHETIC NERVOUS SYSTEM** the part of the autonomic nervous system that is concerned with preparing the body to react to situations of stress or emergency; includes nerves and ganglia

**TENSION MYOSITIS SYNDROME** a disorder involving a painful but harmless change of state in the body's musculature; often attributed to emotional distress

**TRAVELER'S DIARRHEA** a case of dysentery picked up in a foreign country, usually from some unfamiliar bacteria in the local water supply

**TRYPSIN** an enzyme secreted by the pancreas that helps digest proteins

**ULCERATIVE COLITIS** an inflammatory bowel disease in which the inner layer of the colon wall is damaged; associated with abdominal pain, bloody diarrhea, fever, and weight loss

**UPPER ESOPHAGEAL SPHINCTER** an area of high pressure at the end of the pharynx that relaxes to allow swallowed food to enter the esophagus

**WATER BRASH** salty-tasting salivary secretions stimulated by gastroesophageal reflux

**WHEAT INTOLERANCE** a condition in which people suffer unpleasant reactions after consuming wheat or substances containing the wheat protein gluten

# Resources

## Books

James F. Balch, M.D., and Phyllis A. Balch. *Prescription for Nutritional Healing: A Practical A–Z Reference to Drug-Free Remedies Using Vitamins, Minerals, Herbs and Food Supplements.* New York: Avery, 1997.

Norman Cousins. *Anatomy of an Illness.* New York: Bantam Doubleday Dell, 1979.

James Duke. *The Green Pharmacy,* Emmaus, Pa.: Rodale Press, 1997.

Henry D. Janowitz, M.D. *Indigestion: Living Better With Upper Intestinal Problems from Heartburn to Ulcers and Gallstones.* New York: Oxford University Press, 1994.

———. *Your Gut Feelings: A Complete Guide to Living Better With Intestinal Problems.* New York: Oxford University Press, 1994.

Michael Oppenheim, M.D. *The Complete Book of Better Digestion: A Gut-Level Guide to Gastric Relief.* Emmaus, Pa.: Rodale Press, 1990.

Steven Peikin, M.D. *Gastrointestinal Health.* New York: HarperCollins, 1992.

Alan Pressman, D.C., and Donna Shelley, M.D. *Integrative Medicine: The Patient's Essential Guide to Conventional and Complemen-*

*tary Treatments for More Than 300 Common Disorders.* New York: St. Martin's Press, 2000.

*Rome II: The Functional Gastrointestinal Disorders,* 2nd Edition. Edited by Douglas A. Drossman, M.D. (senior editor). McLean, Va.: Degnon, 2000.

John E. Sarno, M.D. *The Mindbody Prescription: Healing the Body, Healing the Pain.* New York: Time Warner, 1998.

W. Grant Thompson, M.D. *The Ulcer Story: The Authoritative Guide to Ulcers, Dyspepsia, and Heartburn.* New York: Plenum Press, 1996.
————. *Gut Reactions: Understanding Symptoms of the Digestive Tract.* New York: Plenum Press, 1989.

David A. Tomb, M.D. *Growing Old: A Complete Guide to the Physical, Emotional, and Financial Problems of Aging.* New York: Viking, 1984.

Andrew Weil, M.D. *Spontaneous Healing.* New York: Ballantine, 1995.

## Web Sites

www.drkoop.com

This site follows the vision of Dr. C. Everett Koop, former U.S. surgeon general, and provides users with comprehensive health-care information. Featured sections include diabetes, clinical trials, multiple sclerosis, and cancer. Visit and learn how to make informed medical decisions and how to reduce your risk factors.

www.webmd.com

Serves all aspects of the health-care industry, from consumers to medical professionals. Teaches users how to stay healthy and how to cope with newly diagnosed illnesses. Provides doctors with tools to improve efficiency and quality. Find out the latest health news, and ask experts questions during live chat events.

www.thedailyapple.com

Access lab-test results, read about your medications, learn

how to assess your health condition, and receive a personalized plan to improve your overall health. In addition, includes access to thousands of health-related articles and studies.

www.health.harvard.edu

The doctors of Harvard Medical School will give you all the information you need to stay healthy. Learn such things as the potentially serious interactions or complications among commonly prescribed medications, drugs, and herbs; how to calculate your body mass index; whether you are at risk for cancer; and what to expect when you need a CAT scan or other diagnostic tests.

www.intelihealth.com

Provides credible information and useful tools on health areas ranging from allergies and headaches to AIDS and stroke. Includes special sections on children's and seniors' health, a drug search, and a medical dictionary.

## Organizations

American Celiac Society—
Dietary Support Coalition
59 Crystal Avenue
West Orange, NJ 07052
(973) 325-8837

Celiac Disease Foundation
13251 Ventura Boulevard, #3
Studio City, CA 91604
(818) 990-2354

Celiac Sprue Association/USA, Inc.
P.O. Box 31700
Omaha, NE 68131-0700
(402) 558-0600

Crohn's and Colitis Foundation of America, Inc.
386 Park Ave. South, 17th Floor
New York, NY 10016-7374
(800) 343-3637; www.ccfa.org
Provides books, newsletters, and brochures about Crohn's disease and ulcerative colitis. Publications may be ordered via telephone. Organizes seminars, medical forums, and public awareness forums. Can refer patients to physicians and self-help groups.

International Foundation for Functional Gastrointestinal
  Disorders
P.O. Box 17864
Milwaukee, WI 53217
(888) 964-2001; www.iffgd.org
Offers fact sheets on gastrointestinal disorders; publishes quarterly newsletter. Annual membership (including newsletter) as of 2001 is $25.

Intestinal Disease Foundation
1323 Forbes Ave., Suite 200
Pittsburgh, PA 15219
(412) 261-5888
Offers information and educational materials on irritable bowel syndrome and other functional disorders, Crohn's disease, colitis, and diverticular disease. Publishes quarterly newsletter and has telephone support program. Annual membership as of 2001 is $25.

National Digestive Diseases Information Clearinghouse
National Institute of Diabetes and Digestive and Kidney
  Diseases
National Institutes of Health
2 Information Way
Bethesda, MD 20892-3570
(301) 654-3810; www.niddk.nih.gov
Provides information on digestive diseases and answers questions.

# Index